THE
☩DANIEL
PLAN

Study Guide + Streaming Video
Six Sessions

BY RICK WARREN
AND THE DANIEL PLAN TEAM

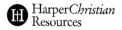

HarperChristian
Resources

The Daniel Plan Study Guide
Copyright © 2013 by The Daniel Plan

Requests for information should be addressed to:
HarperChristian Resources, 3900 Sparks Dr. SE, Grand Rapids, Michigan 49546

978-0-310-15824-0 (softcover)
978-0-310-15825-7 (ebook)

Cover art direction: Curt Diepenhorst
Cover design: Dual Identity
Book Design: Tommy Owen
Contributing Photographers: the PICS Ministry at Saddleback Church, Christopher Broek, Dillon Phommasa, Kent Cameron, Tommy Hyuynh; all other images are courtesy of iStockphoto.

First printed October 2022 / Printed in the United States of America

TABLE OF CONTENTS

A WORD FROM PASTOR RICK

Getting healthy is a choice, and following The Daniel Plan will move you toward living the kind of lifestyle God intends for you to live. I'm so glad you've made this decision because being healthy will impact every area of your life, including your walk with God. The Bible teaches that the starting point for change is dedicating your body to God.

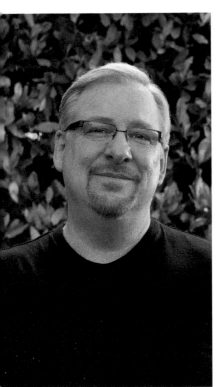

"Therefore, I urge you, brothers and sisters, in view of God's mercy, to offer your bodies as living sacrifices, holy and pleasing to God, this is your spiritual act of worship" (Romans 12:1, NIV). For change to happen in any area of your life—whether you want it to be financial, vocational, educational, mental, relational—it actually works best to begin with the physical. You commit your body to God and all other things follow.

Your health will improve gradually, but you will see consistent change as you stick with The Daniel Plan. What I want you to understand, and I've had to learn this myself, is that you didn't get into the shape you are in now overnight. And so you're not going to get into shape overnight. Just like any form of growth, this is a process, and we've designed The Daniel Plan to keep you engaged in the process so that you will see long-term, lasting results. The Daniel Plan is a lifestyle change that will leave you feeling better and more energetic than you have felt in years.

Here's a guarantee for you: God finishes what he starts. One of the great promises of the Bible is Philippians 1:6 (NLT): "I am sure that God, who began the good work within you, will continue his work until it is finally finished on that day when Christ Jesus comes back again." God is not finished with you. He will be faithful to complete what he has started in you, and he will be faithful to help you complete what you start here ... because what you are doing is dedicating your body to God. As you take these steps, I pray he will bless you in every area of your life.

Rick Warren | Pastor of Saddleback Church | Founder of The PEACE Plan

USING THIS STUDY GUIDE

OUTLINE OF EACH SESSION

Over the next six weeks, you'll gather with friends in a small group to study the Five Essentials of The Daniel Plan: Faith, Food, Fitness, Focus, and Friends. We'll conclude with a session on Living the Lifestyle—practical help on sustaining the healthy changes you've made.

Each group session will include the following:

COMING TOGETHER

The foundation for spiritual growth is an intimate connection with God and his family. A few people who really know you and who earn your trust provide a place to experience the life Jesus invites you to live. You'll use this time to check in with other group members, to report praise and progress: things that went well during the week, positive steps you took, progress you made toward your goals. There's no pressure for everyone to answer all the questions—this is just a chance to "warm up," get to know each other better, and cheer each other on.

LEARNING TOGETHER/VIDEO TEACHING SEGMENT

Each lesson in the study guide begins with a video lesson that has an introduction, testimonies, a message from Pastor Rick Warren, and an interview with a health expert. During the teaching and interview segments, group members should take notes in their study guides, filling in the blanks in the outline and writing down any thoughts or questions that come to mind.

GROWING TOGETHER

Here is where you will process as a group the teaching you heard and watched. The focus won't be on accumulating information but on how we should live in light of the Word of God. We want to help you apply the insights from Scripture practically, creatively, and from your heart as well as your head. Discussing the content of the teaching will help group members understand it better and begin to live out what they've learned. At the end of the day, allowing the timeless truths from God's Word to transform our lives in Christ is our greatest aim.

BETTER TOGETHER

It's one thing to know truth—it's another to live it out. Because this study is about changing our lifestyle, actually being healthier, it simply doesn't make sense to only study the ideas. We need to live them out. This section will offer practical next steps—things that people in the group can actually do to put what they've learned into practice. You'll find very specific "next steps" in the area of that week's study, as well as Food and Fitness tips and activities in every session.

The most fulfilling group experiences happen when the group members do something other than just study together. When they gather outside of the normal group setting, whether for a meal or a workout, or just to connect one-on-one, the group goes deeper and its bonds grow stronger. Encourage group members to be specific about what they plan to do each week as next steps, and encourage them to hold each other accountable. Create an atmosphere of fun, encouragement, and positive reinforcement.

PRAYING TOGETHER

We have Jesus' affirmation that every aspect of life can ultimately be measured as a way of fulfilling one or both parts of the "bottom line" commandment: *"The most important one," answered Jesus, "is this: 'Hear, O Israel, the Lord our God, the Lord is one. Love the Lord your God with all your heart and with all your soul and with all your mind and with all your strength.' The second is this: 'Love your neighbor as yourself.' There is no commandment greater than these"* (Mark 12:29-31, NIV). The group session will close with time for personal response to God and group prayer, seeking to keep this crucial commandment before us at all times. Some lessons will have you praying in groups of two or three, and then closing with the whole group. A "benediction" or written prayer is available, which you may choose to use or not. This is a good place to have different group members close in prayer, even when the instructions don't specify.

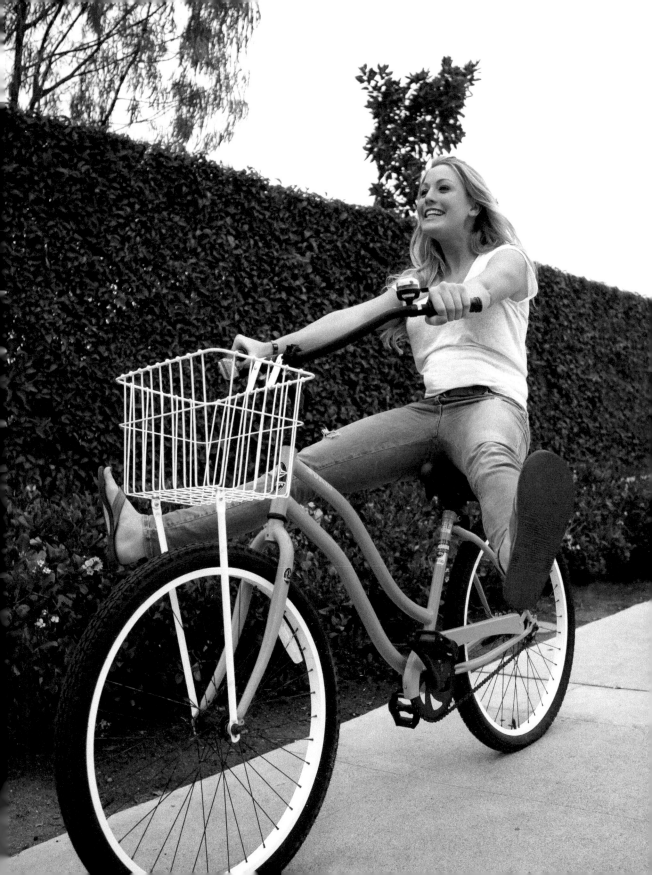

A FEW MORE TIPS

1 Familiarize yourself with the resources in the appendix. Some of them will be used in the sessions themselves.

2 If you are facilitating/leading or co-leading a small group, the section titled Leadership Training 101 will give you some helpful coaching that will enable you to lead well and avoid many common barriers to effective small group leadership.

3 *The Daniel Plan Study Guide* is most effective when used alongside reading *The Daniel Plan: 40 Days to a Healthier Life*. There's a reading guide in the back of this study guide that we hope you'll use. We also recommend that group members access the family of related resources: *The Daniel Plan Journal: 40 Days to a Healthier Life, The Daniel Plan Cookbook: Eating Healthy for Life* and of course The Daniel Plan App and countless free videos and resources on danielplan.com.

4 This study guide is intended to be a flexible resource. If the group responds to the lesson in an unexpected but authentic way, go with that. Let the Holy Spirit lead you. If you think of a better question than the next one in the lesson, ask it. Use the coaching provided in the Frequently Asked Questions pages and the Small Group Resources section.

5 We hope that as you study, you'll linger on the many Scriptures included in each lesson. Faith is the foundation of The Daniel Plan. Encourage group members to pick a verse each week and try memorizing it. Also encourage them to read *The Daniel Plan: 40 Days to a Healthier Life*, and to use *The Daniel Plan Journal: 40 Days to a Healthier Life*, which contain devotionals and more Scriptures to encourage them along the way.

6 We also recommend that you rotate host homes on a regular basis and let the hosts lead the meeting. We've learned that healthy groups rotate leadership. This helps to develop every member's ability to shepherd a few people in a safe environment. Even Jesus gave others the opportunity to serve alongside him (Mark 6:30-44). Look at the FAQs and Leadership 101 pages in the appendix for additional information about hosting or leading the group.

MAKING THE MOST OF THIS STUDY

Take a moment now to complete the 5 Essentials Survey (see appendix). This is your starting point. We all have different starting points, so don't compare yours to anyone else's. This is your unique journey. At the end of this study, on day 40, you will take the survey again and celebrate as you realize all the progress you have made!

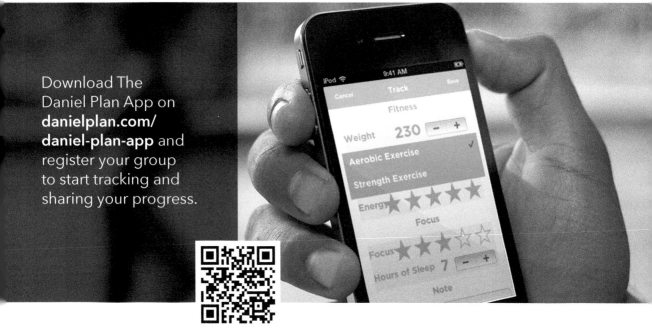

Download The Daniel Plan App on **danielplan.com/daniel-plan-app** and register your group to start tracking and sharing your progress.

EACH WEEK

We highly encourage you to read a few chapters of *The Daniel Plan: 40 Days to a Healthier Life* as you go through this study. This week, read chapters 1–3: How It All Began, The Essentials, and Faith.

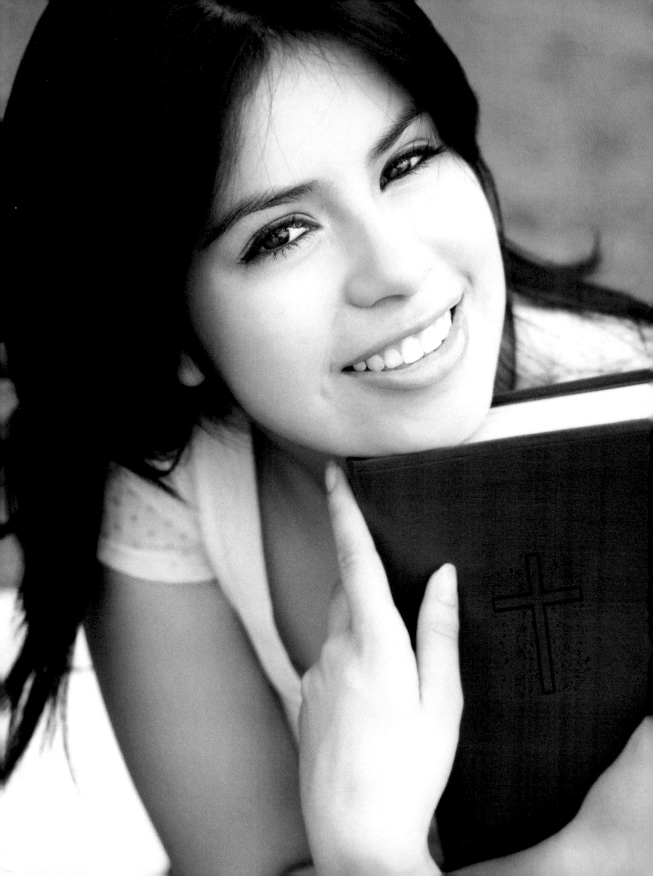

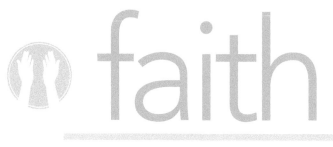

faith

NURTURING *your* SOUL

> "I can do all things
> through Christ who
> strengthens me."
> Philippians 4:13 (WEB)

Many of us are disciplined when it comes to spiritual practices like reading our Bible or going to church, but we may not have that same discipline when it comes to caring for our physical health. Others are careful about eating habits, but ignore caring for the soul. But our spiritual health and physical well-being are intimately connected— and each can strengthen the other. This week, we'll introduce you to the five Essentials of The Daniel Plan, focusing on Faith and its impact on our overall health.

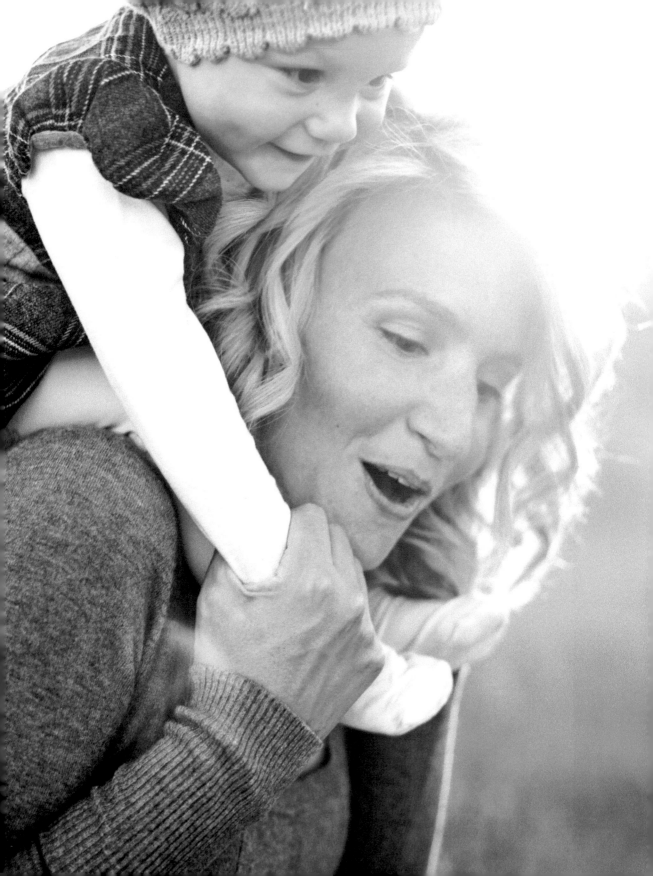

COMING
TOGETHER

In this first section, everyone will have the opportunity to evaluate their starting point for the study, and pick one area of health they would like to focus on for the next six weeks. Since this is the first meeting, go around the room and make sure everyone knows each other's name.

Before you begin, use the Small Group Roster in the appendix to get everyone's contact information. Ask someone to type up the list and email it to everyone in the group this week.

Also, you'll need some simple group guidelines that outline values and expectations. Use the sample in the appendix and make sure that everyone agrees with and understands those expectations.

Use the questions on the following page to start your discussion:

1 The Daniel Plan is a journey toward better health in five essential areas of life. How healthy do you feel in each of these areas, compared to a year ago?

	NOT WELL AT ALL	SOME GOOD DAYS	IMPROVING	MAKING GOOD PROGRESS	DOING GREAT
Faith	1	2	3	4	5
Food	1	2	3	4	5
Fitness	1	2	3	4	5
Focus	1	2	3	4	5
Friends	1	2	3	4	5

2 Pick one of the five Essentials where you'd like to experience positive changes over the next six weeks. What, specifically, are you hoping for in this area of your life?

LEARNING
TOGETHER

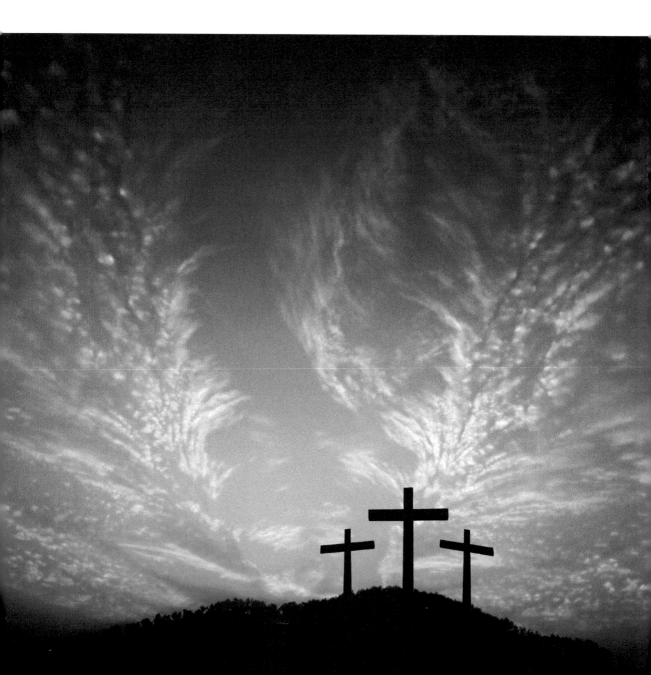

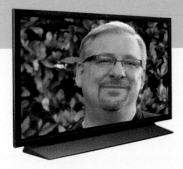

A MESSAGE FROM

Pastor Rick

Watch the video together. Use the following outline to take notes. The answers are in the appendix if you need them.

1 Life is a battle, because everything in the world is _____.

"I don't understand myself at all, for I really want to do what is right, but I can't. I do what I don't want to—what I hate. I know perfectly well that what I am doing is wrong, and my bad conscience proves that I agree with these laws I am breaking. But I can't help myself because I'm no longer doing it. It is sin inside me that is stronger than I am that makes me do these evil things."
Romans 7:15–17 (LB)

"No matter which way I turn I can't make myself do right. I want to but I can't. When I want to do good, I don't; and when I try not to do wrong, I do it anyway."
Romans 7:18-19 (LB)

"My new life tells me to do right, but the old nature that is still inside me loves to sin. Oh, what a terrible predicament I'm in! Who will free me from my slavery to this deadly lower nature? Thank God! It has been done by Jesus Christ our Lord. He has set me free."
Romans 7:23-25 (LB)

"If you are in Christ there is no condemnation for your life."
- Pastor Rick -

Romans chapter 8 gives us six wonderful benefits of _____ in God's Spirit.

"So there is now no condemnation awaiting those who belong to Christ Jesus. For the power of the life-giving Spirit—and this power is mine through Christ Jesus—has freed me from the vicious circle of sin and death."
Romans 8:1-2 (LB)

» All change starts with _____.

» The second thing that helps us to change is the _____.

"Following after the Holy Spirit leads to life and peace, but following after the old nature leads to death."
Romans 8:6 (LB)

"You are controlled by your new nature if you have the Spirit of God living in you."
Romans 8:9 (LB)

"So, dear brothers, you have no obligation, whatever, to your old sinful nature."
Romans 8:12 (LB)

"We are saved by trusting. And trusting means looking forward to getting something we don't yet have—for a man who already has something doesn't need to hope and trust that he will get it. But if we must keep trusting God for something that hasn't happened yet, it teaches us to wait patiently and confidently. And in the same way—by our faith—the Holy Spirit helps us with our daily problems and in our praying."
Romans 8:24-26 (LB)

» We do this by _____.

"And we know that all that happens to us is working for our good if we love God and are fitting into his plans."
Romans 8:28a (LB)

» God will work all for _____.

"What can we ever say to such wonderful things as these? If God is on our side, who can ever be against us? Since he did not spare even his own Son for us but gave him up for us all, won't he also surely give us everything else?"
Romans 8:31–32 (LB)

» God wants you to _____ in your life.

"For I am convinced that nothing can ever separate us from his love. Death can't, and life can't. The angels won't, and all the powers of hell itself cannot keep God's love away. Our fears for today, our worries about tomorrow, or where we are—high above the sky, or in the deepest ocean—nothing will ever be able to separate us from the love of God demonstrated by our Lord Jesus Christ when he died for us."
Romans 8:38–39 (LB)

» God's _____ will never stop.

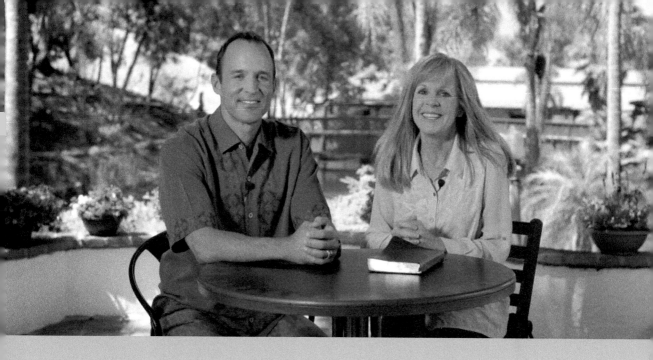

Jimmy Peña Founder of Prayfit

3 _____ is the foundation of The Daniel Plan because faith is the foundation of every part of our lives.

» True faith motivates us to do God's will.

» God's Word provides important tools for overcoming obstacles in our lives.

4 Grace removes the burden of trying to _____ a body that won't last, and yet grace is the reason to honor it, every day that it does.

» It's not about the mirror; it's about the one we're trying to mirror.

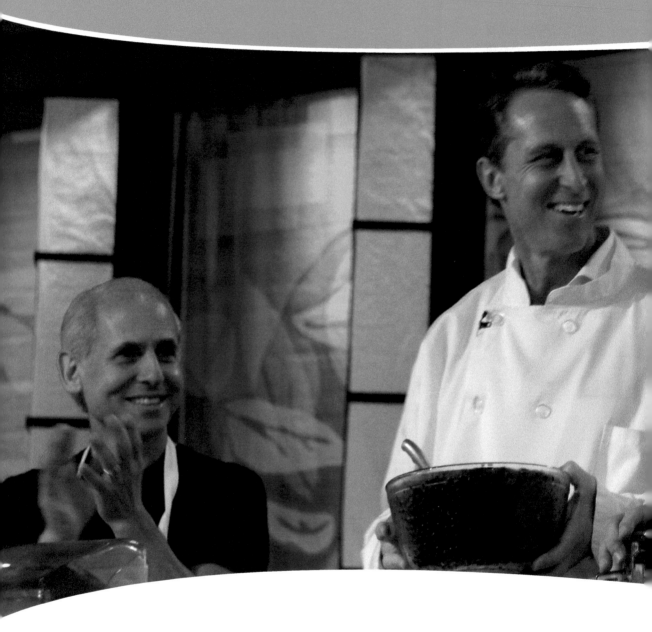

5 Our health is about _____.

» That's the focus of The Daniel Plan: harnessing God's Word, spending time with it every day, and setting the tone for an abundant life.

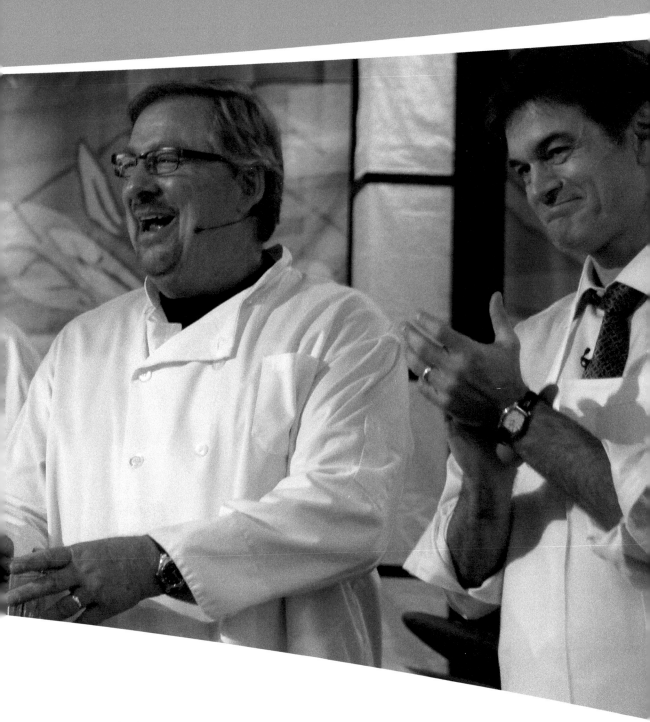

"Therefore, honor God with your bodies."
1 Corinthians 6:20b (NIV)

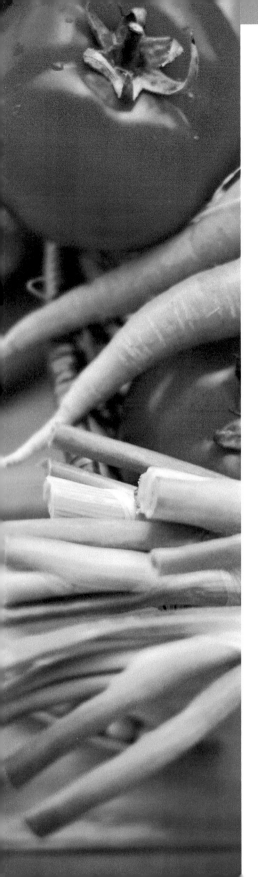

GROWING
TOGETHER

In this section, discuss what you learned from the video teaching. There's no single "right answer" here—just a chance for people to share their stories and listen to each other.

1 Pastor Rick talked about Paul's struggle against his sinful nature, which he writes honestly about in Romans 7. Which of the five Essentials (Faith, Food, Fitness, Focus, or Friends) comes to mind when you read Romans 7: knowing what to do but not doing it?

_____

_____

_____

_____

_____

_____

2   Many of us wrestle with shame—feeling condemned or not good enough. If the Bible says that we have no condemnation, what does that mean to you personally?

_____

_____

_____

_____

3   Jimmy talked about the truth that grace means we don't have to be perfect. Have you ever wrestled with perfectionism? If so, how has that impacted your relationships with God and others?

_____

_____

_____

_____

> _"My son, pay attention to what I say; turn your ear to my words. Do not let them out of your sight; keep them within your heart; for they are life to those who find them and health to one's whole body."_
> Proverbs 4:20–22 (NIV)

In the next section, called Better Together, we will offer you practical next steps to explore what you have learned and apply it to your everyday life. This week we will offer next steps for The Daniel Plan Essential of Faith, along with Food and Fitness tips and recommendations.

BETTER
TOGETHER

Let's get practical—and put what we're learning into action. This week, we're talking about Faith, so be sure you're reaching out and sharing what you are learning about God's truths and promises! We also have Food and Fitness activities for you to choose from.

We have terrific resources to help you on your Daniel Plan journey. Each group member can go to danielplan.com and set up a FREE Daniel Plan Health Profile to track their progress and download The Daniel Plan App with recipes, exercises, and social tools to connect with each other.

Journaling is a great tool for nurturing your faith. *The Daniel Plan Journal: 40 Days to a Healthier Life* helps you track your progress and includes short encouraging devotionals to motivate and inspire you.

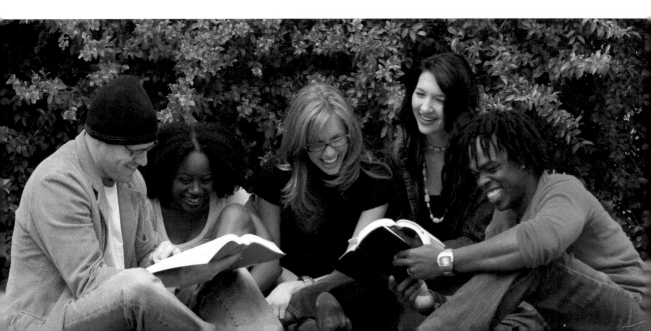

FAITH NEXT STEPS

☐ Pair up with one other person in the group. This will be your spiritual and encouragement partner for the study, your new Daniel Plan buddy. We have learned that people who do The Daniel Plan with another person or a group lose 50 percent more weight! Commit to checking in with each other throughout the week. Even a short text of encouragement is a loving way to let your buddy know you care. Now each of you answer this question: What are you hoping God will do during the next six weeks of this study? After sharing, pray briefly for each other.

☐ Based on your conversation and prayer, select one of the verses from this week's study that you think would be particularly encouraging to your partner. Share that verse with them by writing it on a card for them, or texting it to them. Call or text each other at least once during the week, and pray for each other during the week.

☐ Pick a Bible verse from any part of today's lesson. Write it down, and then read it every day. Try memorizing it and sharing with the group next time. Consider taking on this challenge: memorizing one verse each week during the six weeks of the study.

Here are a few tips and suggested activities to help you move forward on your journey toward health. **Check one or two boxes** next to the options you'd like to try–choose what works for you! You'll find helpful bonus material on the video.

FOOD NEXT STEPS

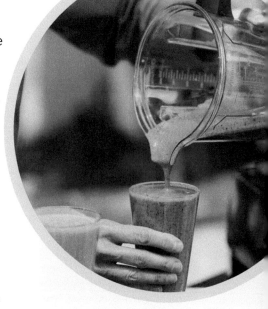

☐ **Food Tip of the Week:** A great way to start your Daniel Plan lifestyle is to clean out your pantry. Click on the QR code to watch a video and learn how, or go to danielplan.com/videos/clean-your-pantry.

☐ **Recipe of the Week:** Learn how easy it is to make a delicious breakfast smoothie. Just click The Daniel Plan Recipe of the Week button on the screen, scan the QR code, or go to danielplan.com/videos/breakfast-smoothie.

☐ **Group Activity of the Week:** Watch the videos together, and then make plans with one or two other group members to clean out your pantries. Help each other get ready to begin a healthy Daniel Plan lifestyle.

FITNESS NEXT STEPS

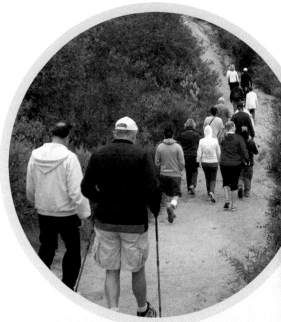

☐ **Fitness Tip of the Week:** The first step in reaching your fitness goals is to believe that you can change. Forget about yesterday, no matter what your attempts to change in the past have been. Today is a new day, and with God's help and power you can do it—one day at a time!

☐ **Move of the Week:** Watch the one-minute Daniel Plan Move of the Week video (just click The Daniel Plan Move of the Week button on the screen). Be adventurous, and try it right now with the group. Or use the QR code, or go to danielplan.com/videos/move-of-the-week to watch it on your own.

☐ **Group Activity of the Week:** Plan an outing with other group members and go for a walk or hike together. If you live near each other, walk in your neighborhood or find a local trail to enjoy.

EACH WEEK

We highly encourage you to read a few chapters of *The Daniel Plan: 40 Days to a Healthier Life* as you go through this study. This week, read chapters 1–3: How It All Began, The Essentials, and Faith.

PRAYING
TOGETHER

Because our efforts at living healthier are strengthened by prayer, we end each meeting with prayer and encourage group members to pray for each other during the week.
This week, try praying this way:

In the large group, simply share your answer to the question, "What are you hoping God will do in your life through this study?" so that others can get to know you and pray for you during the week.

If group members feel comfortable, have a time of prayer in which anyone who would like to pray a short prayer for someone else in the group may do so. The leader can close with the following benediction:

"Father, thank you so much for what you're going to do in our lives. Thank you in advance for giving us the desire to become healthier. We want to get well. We trust that by living out the biblical principles of The Daniel Plan, we will feel better, have more energy, and, Lord willing, live a healthier and longer life. Increase our faith so that we might be a better witness for your glory. We pray this in Jesus' name. Amen."

NOTES

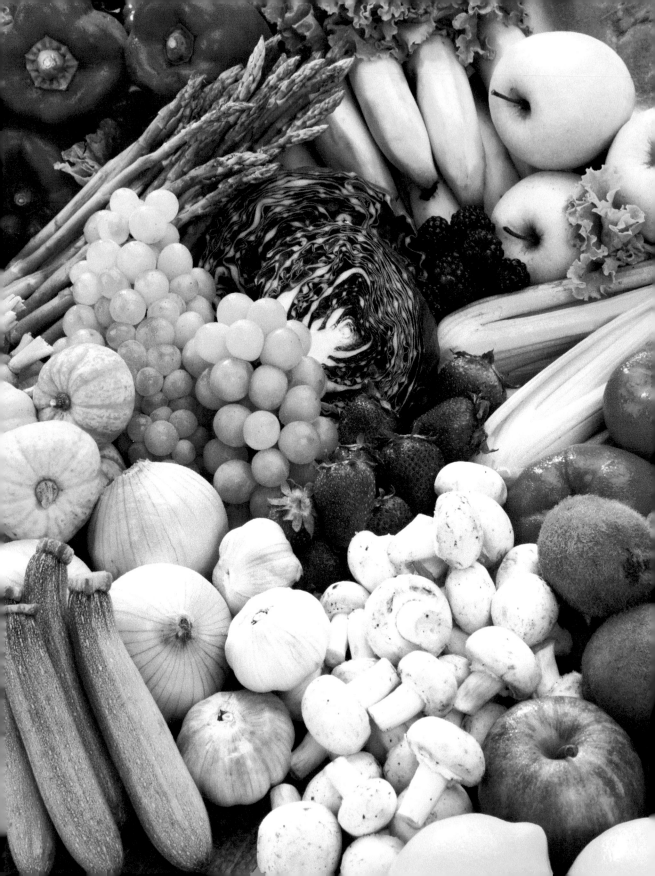

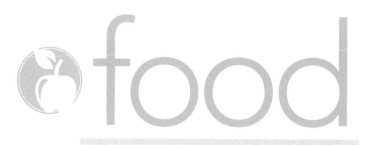

ENJOYING *God's* ABUNDANCE

> "So whether you eat or drink,
> or whatever you do, do it all
> for the glory of God."
> 1 Corinthians 10:31 (NIV)

We are blessed to have an amazing variety of nutrient-rich food available to us. God designed whole food to nourish and fuel our bodies. Although we have many choices, eating well is not as complicated as it might seem. By choosing real foods and avoiding processed and refined products, we begin to experience the healing that good nutrition provides.

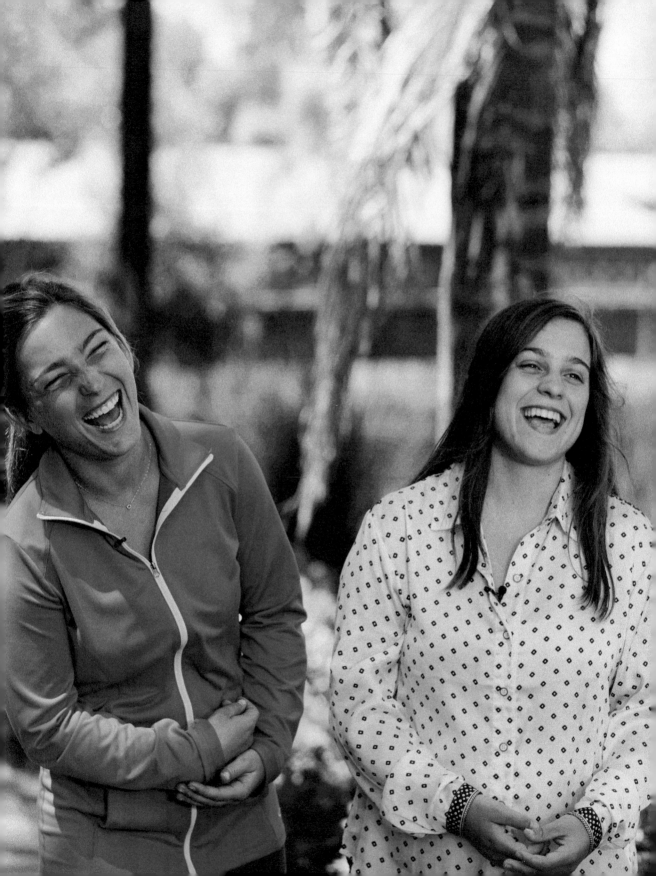

COMING
TOGETHER

1 When you were a kid, what was your favorite food? What memories do you associate with that food or food in general?

_____

_____

_____

2 When you hear the phrase "comfort food," what comes to mind? What is it that is comforting about food?

_____

_____

_____

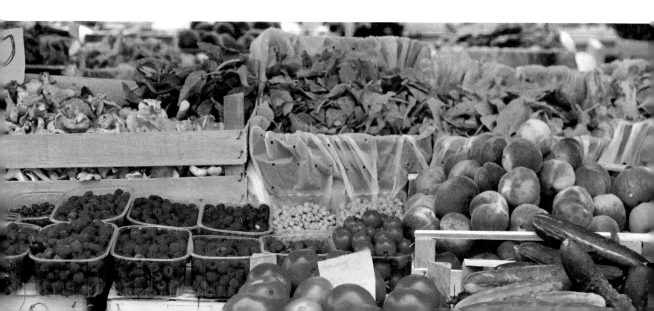

LEARNING
TOGETHER

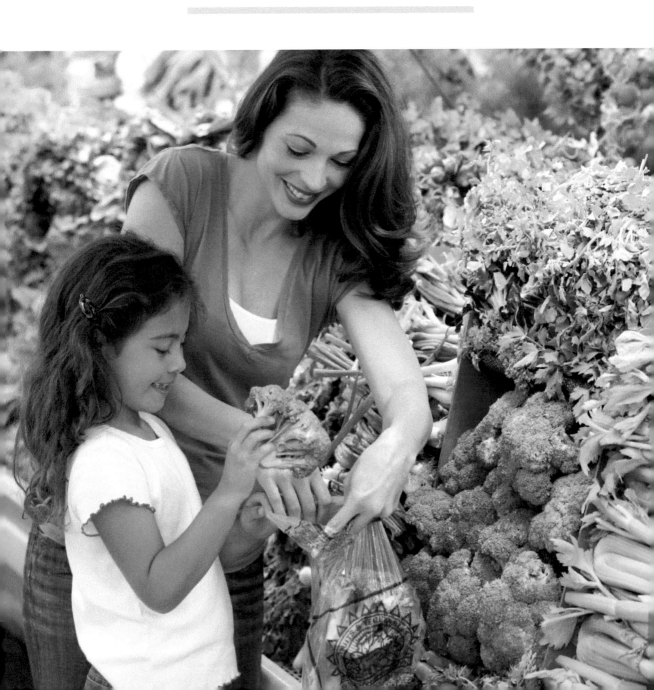

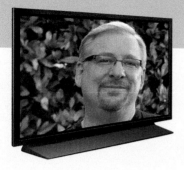

A MESSAGE FROM

Pastor Rick

Watch the video together. Use the following outline to take notes. The answers are in the appendix if you need them.

Nearly 7 out of 10 Americans are _____.

» 80 million people in America are diabetic or pre-diabetic.

» Worldwide, obesity kills as many people as malnutrition.

"'Everything is permissible for me'—but not everything is beneficial. 'Everything is permissible for me'—but I will not be mastered by anything."
1 Corinthians 6:12 (NIV 1984)

"Food for the stomach and the stomach for food, and God will destroy them both."
1 Corinthians 6:13 (NIV)

Your _____ is the temple of the Holy Spirit.

» Your body is a gift from God.

"Do you not know that your bodies are temples of the Holy Spirit, who is in you, whom you have received from God? You are not your own; you were bought at a price."
1 Corinthians 6:19-20 (NIV)

3 God says that you are to be the _____ of your body.

"It is senseless for you to work so hard from early morning until late at night ... God wants his loved ones to get their proper rest."
Psalm 127:2 (LB)

"Don't be drunk with wine, because that will ruin your life."
Ephesians 5:18 (NIV)

"So whether you eat or drink, or whatever you do, do it all for the glory of God."
1 Corinthians 10:31 (NLT)

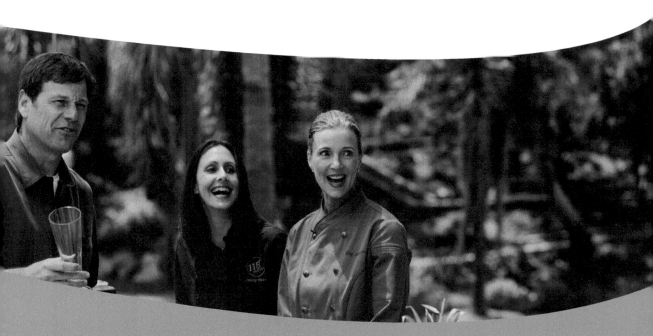

"Let food be thy medicine and thy medicine be food."
- Hippocrates -

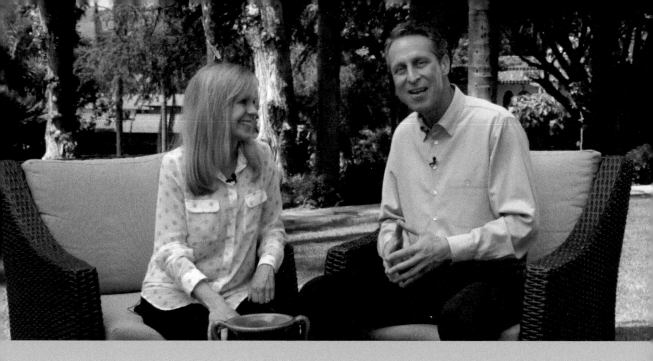

Dr. Mark Hyman

Food isn't just calories and _____; it's actually got _____.

» It's tells your body what to do; it tells it to get sick or to get healthy.

» General rule of thumb: If God made it, it's good for you. If man processed it, it's not good for you.

» The shorter the distance food travels from the field to your fork, the better it is for you.

5 If you do nothing else on The Daniel Plan with food, read your _____ and avoid these 3 things.

» High fructose corn syrup

» Trans fats/hydrogenated fats

» MSG

6 In less than 48 hours, your _____ can completely re-shift.

» Start your day with _____.

» Eat at _____ intervals.

» Don't drink _____-_____ calories.

7 You can eat a lot of food if you eat _____ food.

You're only a couple of days away from feeling good. Give it a try; it's amazing the way you can feel.

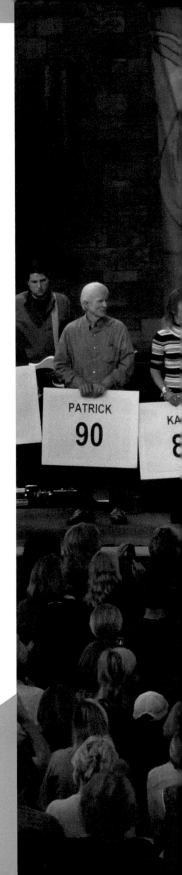

"You cannot exercise your way out of a bad diet."
- Dr. Mark Hyman -

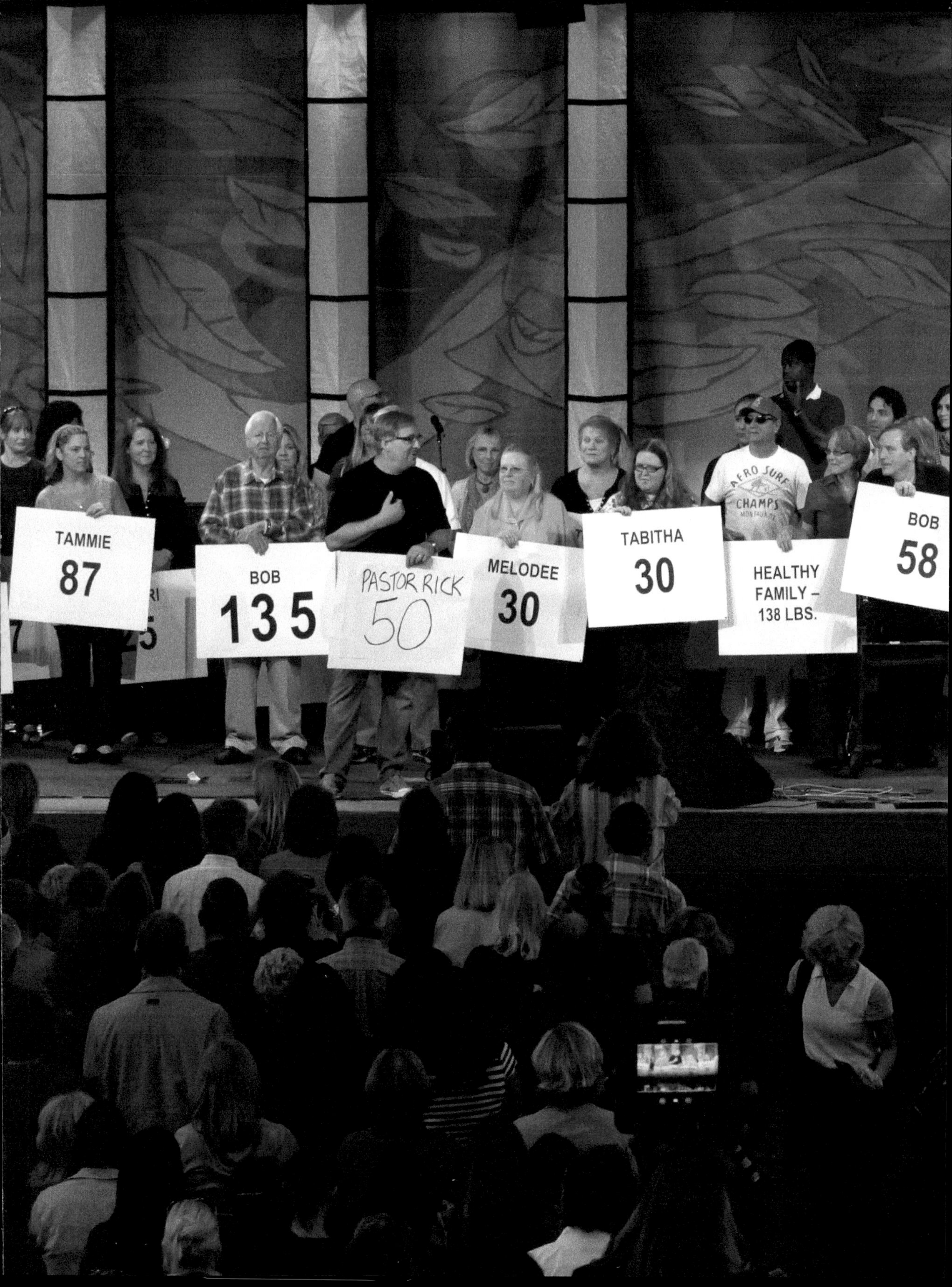

TAMMIE
87

BOB
13 5

PASTOR RICK
50

MELODEE
30

TABITHA
30

HEALTHY
FAMILY –
138 LBS.

BOB
58

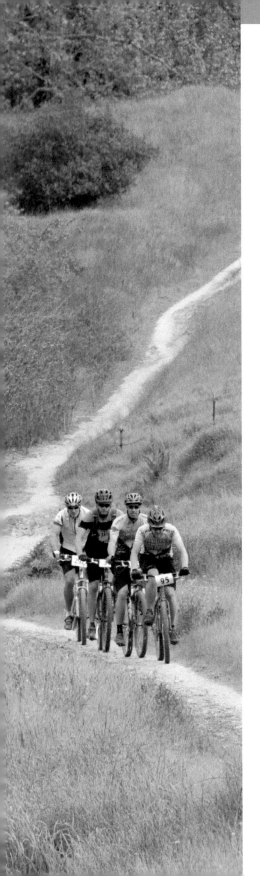

GROWING
TOGETHER

In this section, discuss what you learned from the video teaching. There's no single "right answer" here—just a chance for people to share their stories and listen to each other.

1 In the video, Pastor Rick described his family's dining room table and the dominant place that food had in his family growing up. In what ways is your story similar to, or different from, his?

_____

_____

_____

_____

_____

_____

_____

_____

2 The Bible says that our bodies are temples of God's Spirit and a gift from God. What does that mean to you, on a practical level? What implications does it have for the choices you make?

_____

_____

_____

_____

_____

_____

3 In the video, Dr. Hyman and Dee talked about how you can change your brain in 48 hours based on what you eat. Out of the three things Dr. Hyman suggests, which one would you consider trying this week and why?

_____

_____

_____

_____

_____

In the next section, called Better Together, we will offer you practical next steps to explore what you have learned and apply it to your everyday life. This week we will offer next steps for The Daniel Plan Food Essential, along with Fitness tips and recommendations.

BETTER
TOGETHER

Let's get practical—and put what we're learning into action. This week, we're talking about Food, so explore ways to apply what you've learned and what you put on your plate! We also have Fitness tips and recommendations for you to choose from.

Do you have a copy of *The Daniel Plan: 40 Days to a Healthier Life?* In it you will find an amazing 40-Day Meal Plan with a harvest of fresh ideas to inspire you in the kitchen. Visit danielplan.com to get your copy today.

Here are a few tips and suggested activities to help you move forward on your journey toward health. **Check one or two boxes** next to the options you'd like to try—choose what appeals to you! You'll find helpful bonus material on the video.

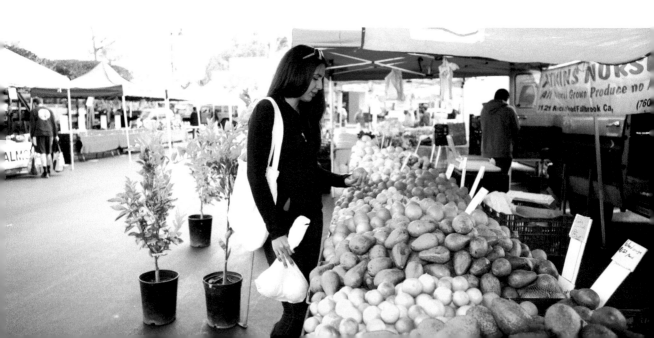

FOOD NEXT STEPS

☐ Food Tip of the Week: Learn to love foods that love you back. Don't let your cravings get the best of you. Read Dr. Hyman's Top 10 Tips to Curb Your Cravings in the appendix.

☐ **Recipe of the Week:** Learn how to create a crowd-stopping taco bar. Just click The Daniel Plan Recipe of the Week button on the screen, scan the QR code, or go to danielplan.com/videos/taco-bar.

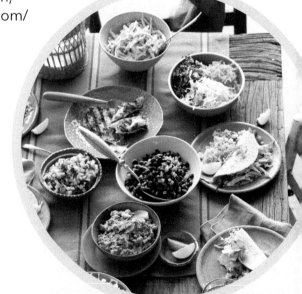

☐ **Group Activity of the Week:** Watch the bonus video to learn how to create a taco bar. Plan a time for the group to meet, have each person bring an ingredient, and enjoy this healthy meal together—perhaps right before your next regularly scheduled meeting.

☐ **Bonus Tip:** Learning what foods to put on your plate is an important step in creating your new eating lifestyle. Get a head start by looking at The Daniel Plan Plate and some suggested foods in the appendix.

Here is The Daniel Plan 3-Day Meal Plan for you to try! Every recipe is simple to make, with ingredients you can find at any store. Feel free to swap out fruit and vegetables based on the season or your tastes. Explore different spices and herbs to add flavor. Bring your family and friends into the kitchen to partake in the creation of meals. When you follow The Daniel Plan approach, cooking food becomes a joy! Scan the QR code or go to danielplan.com/recipes/3-day-meal-plan for all the recipes.

Meal	Day 1	Day 2	Day 3
Breakfast	Dr. Hyman's whole food protein shake	1 c. rolled or steel cut oatmeal with ½ c. almond milk & ½ c. mixed strawberries and bananas	Breakfast wrap: 1 scrambled egg with ¼ avocado, sliced tomato, basil wrapped in whole grain tortilla
Snack	Mixed veggie sticks (celery, carrots, cucumber, jicama) and 1/3 c. artichoke hummus	½ c. mixed berries plus 25 cinnamon toasted almonds	Small apple plus 25 raw almonds
Lunch	½ c. quinoa with steamed broccoli and carrots and antioxidant salad dressing	Grilled citrus salmon with supergreens watermelon salad	Veggie lentil & chicken sausage soup
Snack	Veggie juice mocktail	2 tbsp. crunchy chickpeas with 2 hardboiled eggs	Creamy carrot dip with steamed veggies
Dinner	Thai-inspired stir fry with coconut rice	Crockpot beef and veggie stew	Dr. Hyman's walnut pesto chicken with white beans, chopped peppers, balsamic vinegar

FITNESS NEXT STEPS

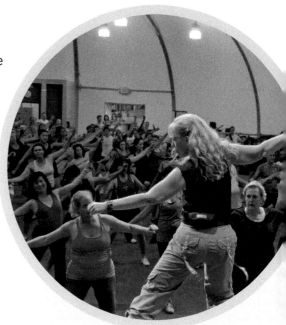

☐ Fitness Tip of the Week: If you have not been exercising lately, the best way to ease back into a regular fitness program is to start with a small step. Set small, realistic goals to make it easy to fit exercise into your daily schedule. You will increase your confidence as you accomplish your goals step by step.

☐ Move of the Week: Watch the one-minute Daniel Plan Move of the Week on the video (just click The Daniel Plan Move of the Week button on the screen). Why not try it right now with the group, use the QR code, or go to danielplan.com/videos/move-of-the-week to watch it on your own.

☐ Group Activity of the Week: Plan an outing with other group members this week to work out together. If you enjoy exercising in a larger group setting, try taking a class you've never done before. Share your experience with the group next week.

EACH WEEK

We highly encourage you to read a few chapters of *The Daniel Plan: 40 Days to a Healthier Life* as you go through this study. This week, read chapters 4 and 10: Food and 40-Day Meal Plan.

PRAYING
TOGETHER

Because our efforts at living healthier are strengthened by prayer, we end each meeting with prayer and encourage group members to pray for each other during the week. This week, try praying this way:

Get into groups of two or three people. Have each person briefly share a challenge they face when it comes to making healthy choices about food—such as feeling tempted by junk food, or finding themselves in a food emergency. Spend some time praying for one another's concerns.

After everyone has had some time to pray, the leader can close with this benediction from Pastor Rick's message:

"Father, you created our body. You sent Jesus to pay for our body and you sent your Spirit to live in our body. Help us to always remember that our body belongs to you. Thank you for giving us food to enjoy and nourish the body you gave us. Forgive us for the many times we have misused our body and abused our health due to an unhealthy diet. As we make healthier choices, change our tastes so our desires become what you would want them to be. As we continue on this journey of health, help us follow your health plan for your glory. In Jesus' name. Amen."

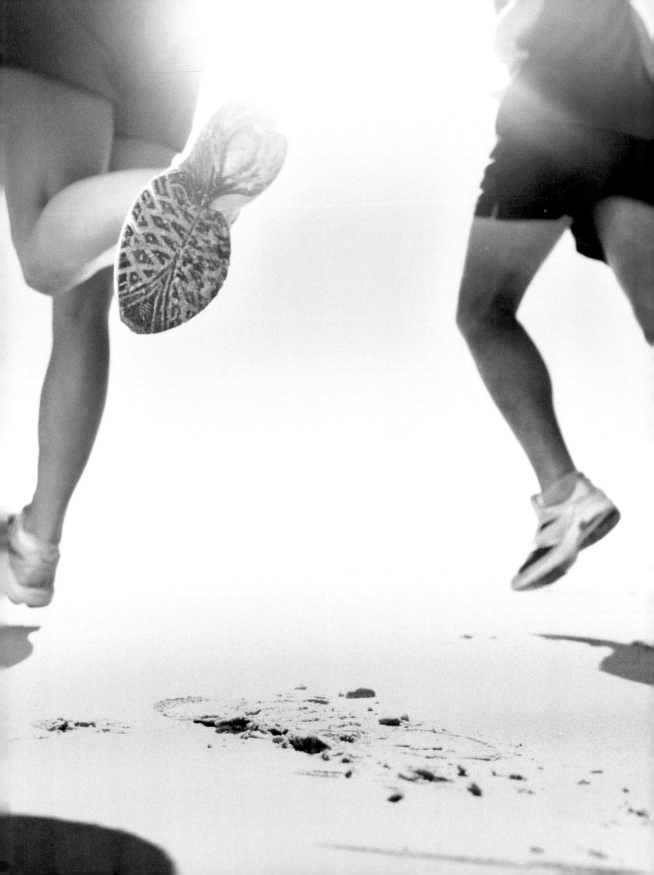

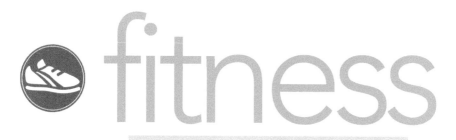

fitness

STRENGTHENING *your* BODY

"Do you not know that your bodies
are temples of the Holy Spirit …
Therefore honor God with
your bodies."
1 Corinthians 6:19a, 20b (NIV)

All of us know that exercise is good
for us: it makes us feel better, gives
us more energy, and can even help
improve the quality of our lives. We
know we "should" exercise, but we
don't do always do it. This week, we
are going to talk not just about the
benefits of exercise but about how to
get motivated and find
movement you enjoy!

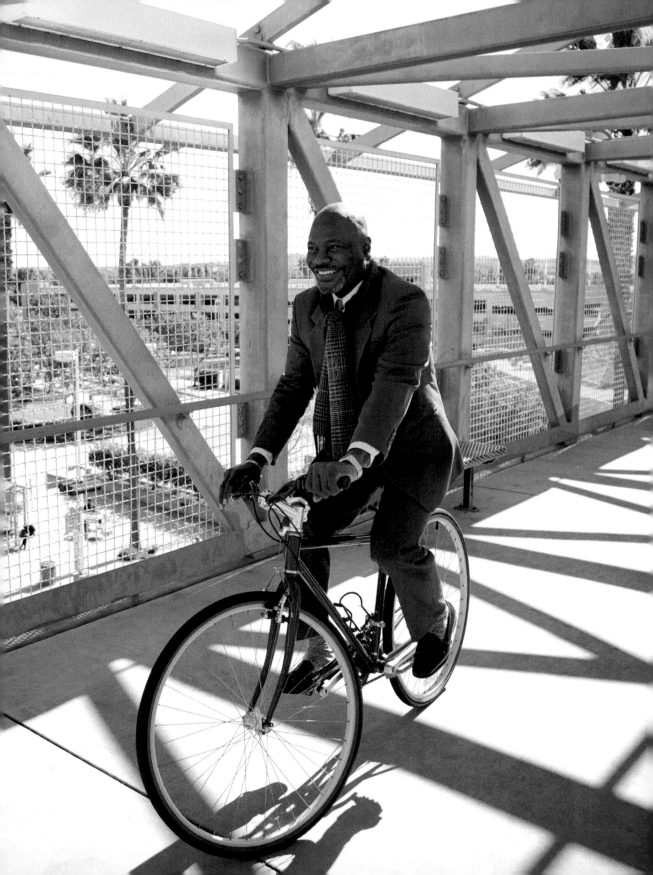

COMING
TOGETHER

Start by sharing and celebrating progress. Did anyone try the move of the week or a new recipe? Did anyone memorize a verse or learn something new? Use these questions to jump-start the conversation.

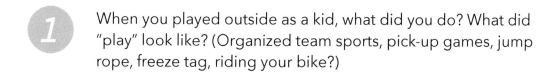

1 When you played outside as a kid, what did you do? What did "play" look like? (Organized team sports, pick-up games, jump rope, freeze tag, riding your bike?)

_____

_____

_____

2 In Chapter 5 of *The Daniel Plan: 40 Days to a Healthier Life*, we find this thought-provoking question: "If I could realize or accomplish anything related to my fitness and health, without fear of failure, what would it be?" How would you answer that question?

LEARNING
TOGETHER

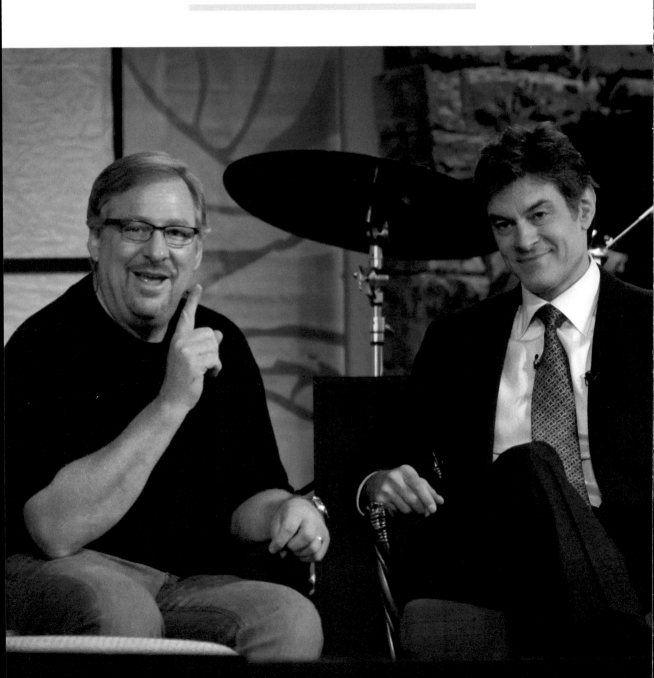

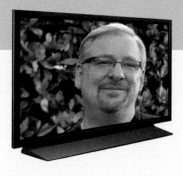

A MESSAGE FROM

Pastor Rick

Watch the video together. Use the following outline to take notes. The answers are in the appendix if you need them.

1 The Bible tells us, in preparing ourselves, we have to _____ our hearts and we have to _____ our bodies.

» I purify my heart by committing my thought life to God.

» I sanctify my body by dedicating my physical body to God's purpose.

"You made my body, Lord; now give me sense to heed your laws."
Psalm 119:73 (LB)

"Therefore, I urge you, brothers and sisters, in view of God's mercy, to offer your bodies as a living sacrifice, holy and pleasing to God—this is your true and proper worship."
Romans 12:1 (NIV)

"It is senseless for you to work so hard from early morning until late at night ... for God wants his loved ones to get their proper rest."
Psalm 127:2 (LB)

"The reason I want you and I to be healthy is because it will give us more energy to do the things God wants us to do."
- Pastor Rick -

2 One-third of Jesus' ministry was helping people get _____ healthy.

» Jesus cares about your mind and your body–your overall HEALTH!

3 The Bible advises us to _____ our body.

"Do you not know that your bodies are temples of the Holy Spirit, who is in you, whom you have received from God? You are not your own; you were bought at a price. Therefore honor God with your bodies."
1 Corinthians 6:19–20 (NIV)

When you love God, and you love other people, then your
_____ for being healthy changes.

> » God has promised to bless goals, when you commit your body to him.

> » For change to happen, it actually works best to begin with the physical.

 Caring for your body is an act of _____. It is also an act of
_____.

> » What you think you own is really on loan.

> *"No one hates his own body but feeds and cares for it, just as Christ cares for the church."*
> Ephesians 5:29 (NLT)

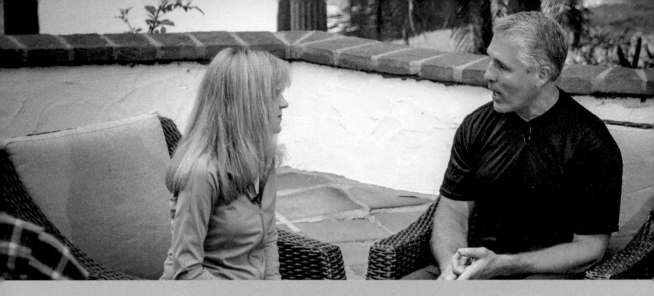

AN INTERVIEW WITH

Sean Foy Exercise Physiologist

The best exercise is the one that you will actually_____.

» Performing simple, 15-30 second movements at your desk a few times a day can significantly improve your health.

» Short bursts of exercise, just three or four times a day, can drastically improve your fitness level.

"Becoming Daniel Strong is the act of pursuing excellence so that we can glorify God physically, emotionally, relationally, and spiritually."

- Sean Foy -

Physical motion affects _____.

» Simple deep breathing exercises and easy stretching movements can significantly improve your health.

» If you can schedule your activity before it happens, it is very beneficial.

» Schedule exercise and track your progress. Use a journal.

» The more you move, the better you will feel. The better you feel, the greater the likelihood that you will exercise more. It's a positive cycle.

"For God's temple is holy, and you are that temple."
1 Corinthians 3:17b (NLT)

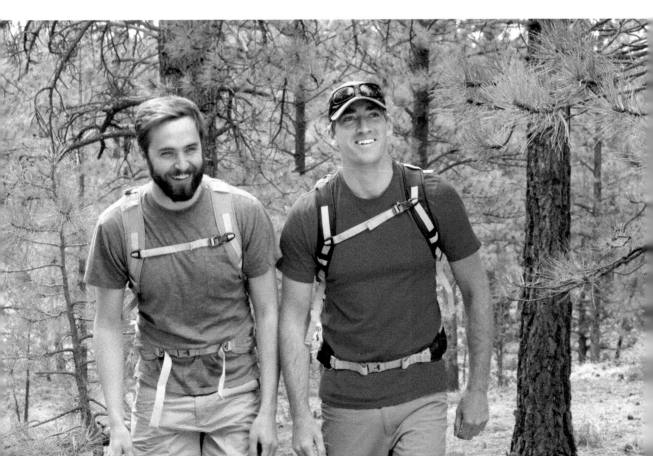

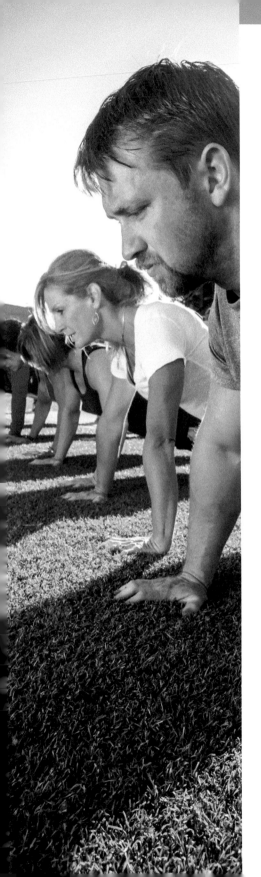

GROWING
TOGETHER

In this section, discuss what you learned from the video teaching. There's no single "right answer" here—just a chance for people to share their stories and listen to each other.

1 Pastor Rick said we typically reject, neglect, perfect, or protect our bodies. Share about a time that one of those words describes how you treated your body. What happened? How did that impact your overall health? What's one thing you could do this week to "protect" your body?

_____

_____

_____

_____

_____

_____

2 The best exercise is actually the one you will do. Share about an exercise you have tried in the past, or something you'd like to consider in the future.

_____

_____

_____

_____

3 Sean talked about getting a buddy to work out with—it might even be your dog! Who is your exercise buddy? If you don't have one, what's one small step you could take to find one?

_____

_____

_____

_____

In the next section, called Better Together, we will offer you practical next steps to explore what you have learned and apply it to your everyday life. This week we will offer next steps for The Daniel Plan Fitness Essential, along with Food tips and recommendations.

BETTER
TOGETHER

Let's get practical—and put what we're learning into action. This week, we're talking about Fitness, so be sure to make plans to try at least one of the suggested activities. You might even want to set a goal to move for 20 minutes every day this week. We also have Food activities for you to choose from.

Here are a few tips and suggested activities to help you move forward on your journey toward health. Check one or two boxes next to the options you'd like to try—choose what works for you! You'll find helpful bonus material on the video.

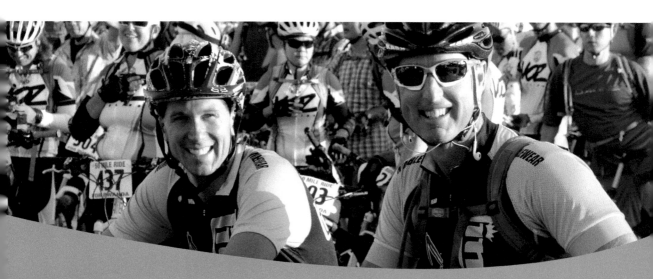

"The best exercise for you is the one you will do and do consistently."
- Sean Foy -

FITNESS NEXT STEPS

☐ **Fitness Tip of the Week:** Choose exercises you enjoy. The best exercise to help you get fit and stay fit is THE ONE YOU WILL DO! Begin with exercises or movements that bring a smile to your face. Consider inviting a friend to join you.

☐ **Move of the Week:** Watch the one-minute Daniel Plan Move of the Week video. Just click The Daniel Plan Move of the Week button on the screen. Try it right now with the group, use the QR code, or go to danielplan.com/videos/move-of-the-week to watch it on your own.

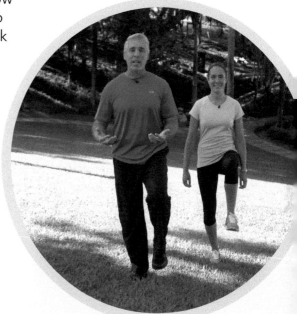

☐ **Group Activity of the Week:** How would you like to rev up your metabolism, burn 200–300 extra calories a day, and get in shape without sweating at all from 9 to 5? Go to danielplan.com for how to add small, simple activities throughout the day that will bring movement into your everyday life.

FOOD NEXT STEPS

☐ **Food Tip of the Week:** A great way to be successful and avoid a food emergency is to plan ahead. Reserve time to pre-cook your protein and cut up veggies for the week. If you missed the video last week from Dr. Hyman on how to avoid a food emergency, scan the QR code, or go to danielplan.com/videos/how-to-avoid-a-food-emergency to watch and learn.

☐ **Recipe of the Week:** Love pasta? We've got good news for you! We've got pasta on your menu this week. Just click The Daniel Plan Recipe of the Week button on the screen, scan the QR code, or go to danielplan.com/videos/pasta.

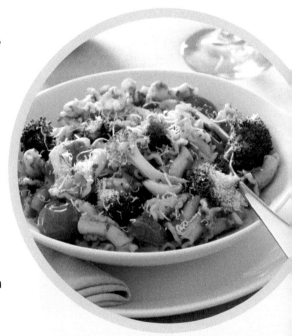

☐ **Group Activity of the Week:** Make plans to go grocery shopping with your buddy from the group—and help each other to make healthy choices. Use the shopping list on danielplan.com to guide you.

EACH WEEK

We highly encourage you to read a few chapters of *The Daniel Plan: 40 Days to a Healthier Life* as you go through this study. This week, read chapters 5 and 9: Fitness and Daniel Strong 40-Day Fitness Challenge.

PRAYING
TOGETHER

Because our efforts at living healthier are strengthened by prayer, we end each meeting with prayer and encourage group members to pray for each other during the week. This week, pray this way:

Get into smaller groups of two or three people. Have each person share the one thing they plan to do this week to "protect" their body—it might be protecting it from junk food or strengthening it by going to an exercise class. Pray together that each of you would take that step toward better health. Agree to pray for each other during the week.

After you've prayed in smaller groups, the leader can close with this benediction from Pastor Rick's message:

"Father, thank you for our body. We know that you gave us our body on loan to take care of it so we can serve you better. Help us to honor you by honoring our body. Teach us how to lovingly care for our body just as Jesus so gently cares for the body of Christ. We want to achieve better health by taking care of our body. We know we can do that when we focus on your Word and your ways. Thank you, God, for creating us just as we are. Amen."

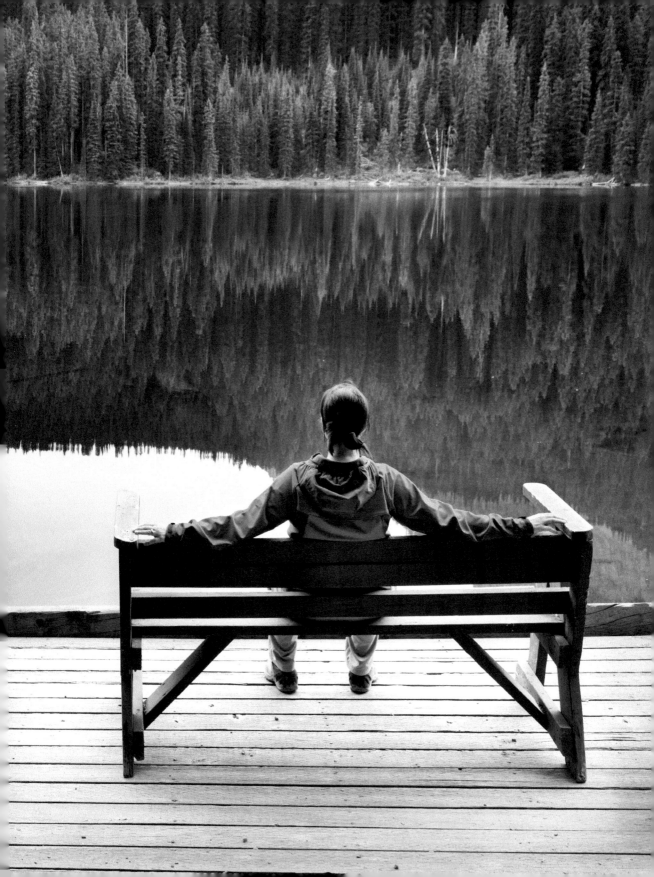

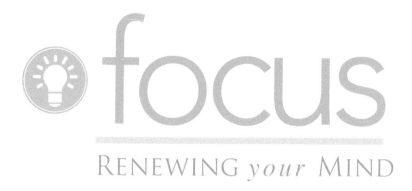

focus

RENEWING *your* MIND

> "Do not conform to the pattern of this world, but be transformed by the renewing of your mind."
> Romans 12:2 (NIV)

Over the past few weeks, you've started to make some changes in the areas of Faith, Food, and Fitness. How do you sustain those changes? How do you accomplish that which is truly important instead of being distracted by things that are urgent? This week, we'll offer you some specific steps to improve your focus—which is the key to long-term, sustainable change.

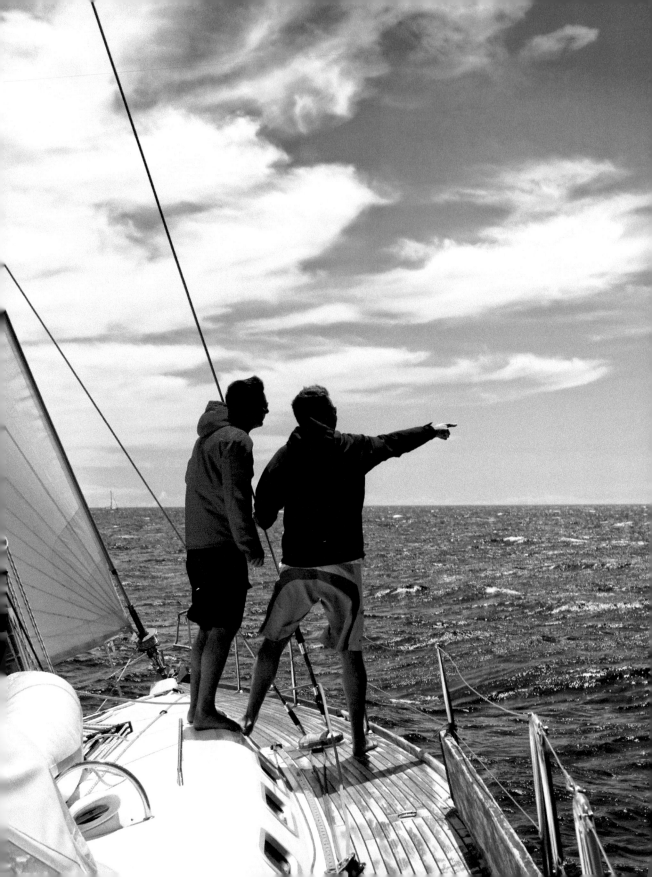

COMING
TOGETHER

Start by sharing and celebrating progress. Did anyone try the move of the week or a new recipe? Did anyone memorize a verse or learn something new? Use these questions to jump-start the conversation.

1 A key to The Daniel Plan is remembering that small steps lead to big results. Share one "small step" success you had on The Daniel Plan this week: one positive step you took or one positive outcome of a choice you made.

_____

_____

_____

_____

_____

_____

_____

_____

2 On a scale of 1 to 10, with 1 being absolutely no stress, and 10 being chronic stress, what is the current stress level in your life and why?

(1) (2) (3) (4) (5) (6) (7) (8) (9) (10)

"Chronic stress constricts blood flow to the brain, which lowers overall brain function and prematurely ages your brain." - Dr. Daniel Amen
- *The Daniel Plan: 40 Days to a Healthier Life, Chapter 6*

3 Based on your experience, how much does stress affect your ability to focus?

LEARNING
TOGETHER

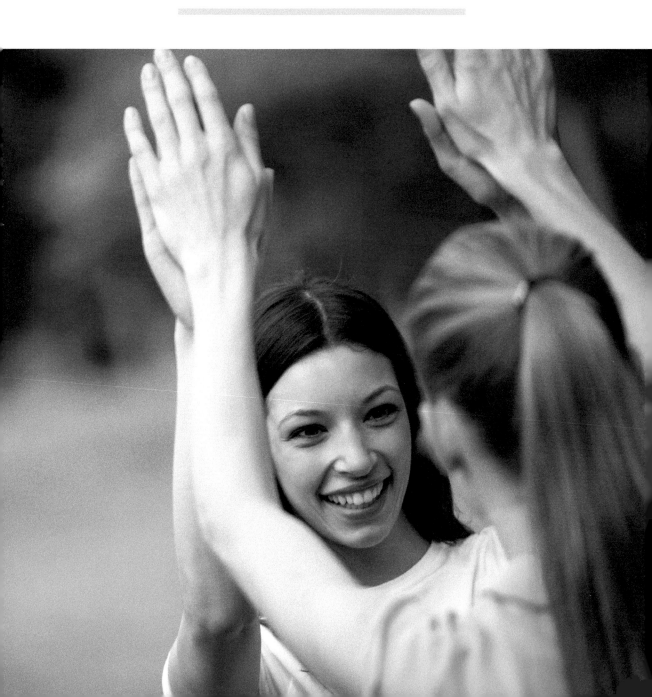

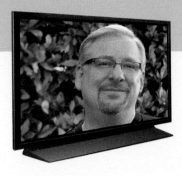

A MESSAGE FROM

Pastor Rick

Watch the video together. Use the following outline to take notes. The answers are in the appendix if you need them.

"Redeeming the time, because the days are evil."
Ephesians 5:16 (NKJV)

 Make a _____.

> » When you share a goal with someone else, your chance of achieving it increases dramatically.

> » Clarify what matters most, calculate the time, and put it on the calendar.

 Be ruthless with _____.

> » Whatever gets your attention gets you.

> » Stop focusing on what you don't want and start focusing on what you do want.

"Do not conform to the pattern of this world, but be transformed by the renewing of your mind."
Romans 12:2 (NIV)

"The secret to an effective life is focus. Don't try to do fifty things that you dabble in. Know what's most important, and do those things—and don't worry about anything else."
- Rick Warren -

Change is always a _____.

» If you change your brain, you can change your life.

» The urgent is almost never the most important thing.

» Goals focus your energy.

 A goal is a dream with a _____.

» A goal is very specific, measurable, and timely.

» Long-term goals keep you from being discouraged by short-term setbacks.

"My counsel is this: Live freely, animated and motivated by God's Spirit. Then you won't feed the compulsions of selfishness."
Galatians 5:16 (MSG)

"May our Lord Jesus Christ himself and God our father who loved us and by his grace gave us eternal encouragement and good hope, encourage your hearts and strengthen you in every good deed and word."
2 Thessalonians 2:16–17 (NIV)

"For it is God who works in you to will and to act in order to fulfill his good purpose."
Philippians 2:13 (NIV)

"For God has not given us a spirit of fear and timidity, but of power, love, and self-discipline."
2 Timothy 1:7 (NLT)

"I pray that from his glorious, unlimited resources he will empower you with inner strength through his Spirit."
Ephesians 3:16 (NLT)

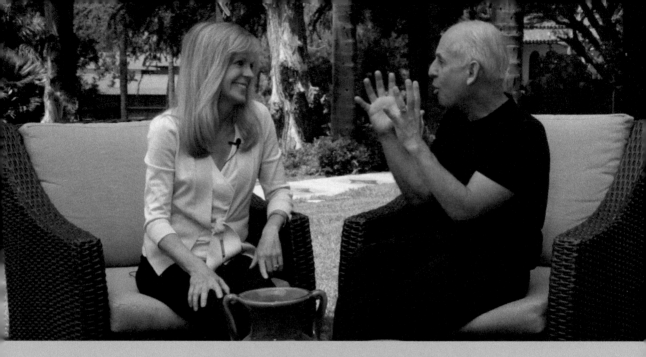

AN INTERVIEW WITH

Dr. Daniel Amen

Emotions drive _____.

» Getting your mind right is such an important pillar to being healthy overall.

» Embrace all five Essentials. All impact your thoughts, and your thoughts impact your health.

» Positive thoughts release positive chemicals in your brain. Negative thoughts release negative chemicals.

Your thoughts sometimes lie! Whenever you feel sad, mad, nervous, or out of control, write down your thought and then ask, "Is it _____?"

» Uninvestigated thoughts can cause stress in our lives.

» Research shows that prayer optimizes brain function.

"Finally, brothers and sisters, whatever is true, whatever is noble, whatever is right, whatever is pure, whatever is lovely, whatever is admirable—if anything is excellent or praiseworthy—think about such things."
Philippians 4:8 (NIV)

 Where you bring your attention determines how you _____.

» Focus on what you are grateful for.

» Turn bad days into good data. On the Daniel Plan you cannot fail, because every failure is really just a lesson to help you.

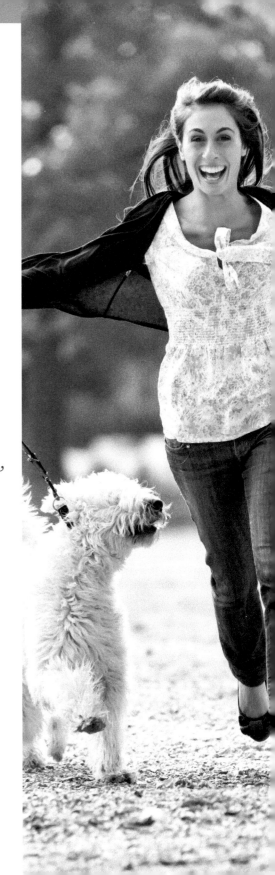

GROWING
TOGETHER

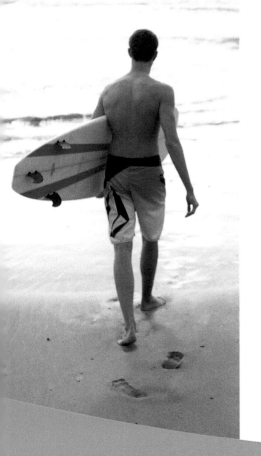

In this section, discuss what you learned from the video teaching. There's no single "right answer" here—just a chance for people to share their stories and listen to each other.

1 In this week's video, Pastor Rick stated, "No matter what kind of change you want to make in your life—mental, physical, financial, spiritual, social, whatever—the key to changing for the better is finding the energy to make that change." Share about a time you made a significant change in your life. What motivated you (that is, where did you find the energy to make that change)?

_____

_____

_____

"The desire and motivation we need to change must ultimately come from God."
- Pastor Rick -

2   Pastor Rick spoke about the wise use of time. He told the story about his peach tree and how he has been throwing away some of his baby "peaches" so his branches don't get weighed down with too much small fruit. What are some of the "good" things in your life (baby fruit) that distract you from doing the most important things?

_____

_____

_____

3   Let's look back at Pastor Rick's and Dr. Amen's suggestions for better overall health and pick one or two that you want to work on this week. What are some specific attitudes or actions you can adopt that will help increase your energy levels?

_____

_____

_____

4   Dr. Amen repeatedly emphasized the importance of focusing on positive thoughts and freeing ourselves of negativity, because where you focus your attention determines how you feel. What circumstances in your life cause you to slip into negativity? What are some biblical truths that could replace negative thoughts?

_____

_____

_____

In the next section, called Better Together, we will offer you practical next steps to explore what you have learned and apply it to your everyday life. This week we will offer next steps for The Daniel Plan Focus Essential, along with Food and Fitness tips and recommendations.

BETTER
TOGETHER

Let's get practical—and put what we're learning into action. This week, we're talking about Focus, so here's an activity that will improve your brain function and emotional well-being. We also have Food and Fitness activities for you to choose from.

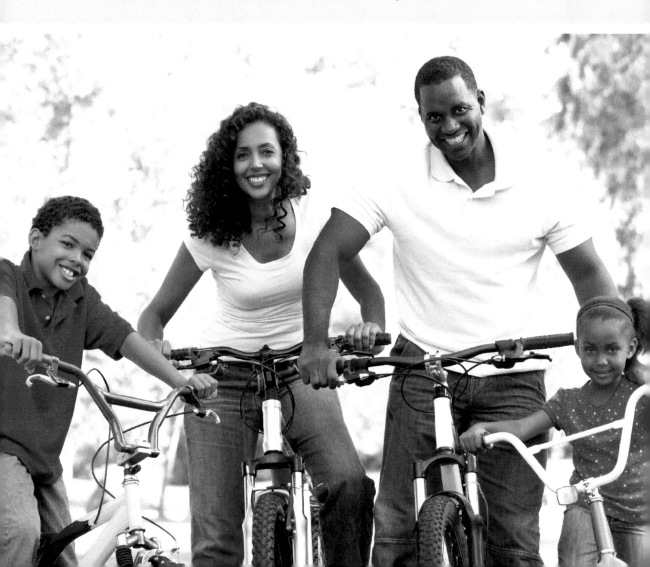

FOCUS NEXT STEPS

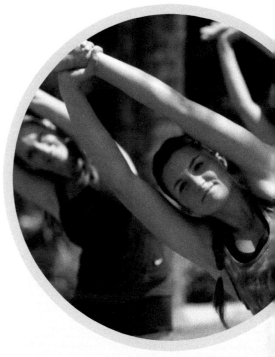

☐ In the space provided below, write down one thing you are grateful for. Just doing so will enhance your brain. Have a few group members share what they've written.

_____

_____

☐ Each day this week, write down three different things for which you are thankful. Notice how this exercise impacts your overall health, your level of optimism, your general mood. You may want to record what you notice in your journal. Share your findings with the group next time you meet.

Need a place to journal your gratitude? *The Daniel Plan Journal: 40 Days to a Healthier Life* is available at **www.danielplan.com/resources**

"The act of writing down your grateful thoughts helps to bring your attention to them to enhance your brain … researchers have found that people who express gratitude on a regular basis are healthier, more optimistic, make more progress toward their goals, have a greater sense of well-being, and they are more helpful to others."

- The Daniel Plan

Here are a few tips and suggested activities to help you move forward on your journey toward health. **Check one or two boxes** next to the options you'd like to try–choose what works for you! You'll find helpful bonus material on the video.

FOOD NEXT STEPS

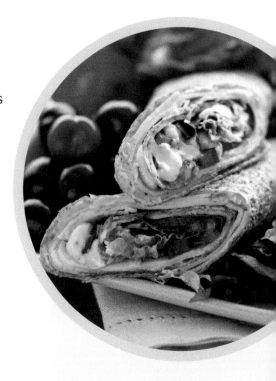

☐ **Tip of the Week:** Set a specific, measurable goal for your eating plan this week. For example: "I will add two more servings of vegetables to my plate each day this week."

☐ **Recipe of the Week:** Daniel Plan-inspired wraps are delicious and nutritious. This week learn how easy it is to make wraps that everyone will enjoy. Just click The Daniel Plan Recipe of the Week button on the screen, scan the QR code, or go to danielplan.com/videos/wrap.

☐ **Group Activity of the Week:** Watch the video to learn how to create a wrap. Ask everyone to get creative and make their version of a tasty wrap and bring it to your next meeting. Just slice them up to share!

FITNESS NEXT STEPS

☐ **Tip of the Week:** Plan your exercise before your week begins: Good exercise habits happen because we make them happen. Schedule appointments with yourself, writing down on your calendar the exact day and time you are committing to move your body.

☐ **Move of the Week:** Watch the one-minute Daniel Plan Move of the Week video (just click The Daniel Plan Move of the Week button on the screen). Why not try it right now with the group, use the QR code, or go to danielplan.com/videos/move-of-the-week to watch it on your own.

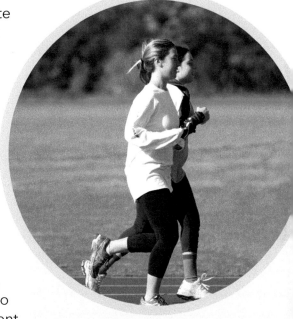

☐ **Group Activity of the Week:** Increase your progress by finding an exercise buddy to work out with you this week. It can be someone from the group, a friend, or family member. Remember, people who do The Daniel Plan together lose 50 percent more weight!

EACH WEEK

We highly encourage you to read a few chapters of *The Daniel Plan: 40 Days to a Healthier Life* as you go through this study. This week, read Chapter 6: Focus.

PRAYING
TOGETHER

Because our efforts at living healthier are strengthened by prayer, we end each meeting with prayer, and encourage group members to pray for each other during the week. This week, pray this way:

Get into groups of two or three people. Have each person briefly share what they plan to do this week to limit distractions. Then have everyone pray for each other, asking God to equip them with his power and strength to achieve this goal.

After everyone has had some time to pray, the leader can close with this benediction from Pastor Rick's message:

"Dear God, we commit our journey to health as an act of worship. Like the Bible says, we want to offer our body and our mind as a living sacrifice, acceptable to you. God, we want nothing more than to be good stewards of our thoughts and feelings. We commit to living a more focused life and we want to begin by reading your Word every day, so our mind will be filled with your truths. We do not want to conform to the world but conform to your Word, so that your promises can become true in our life. God, we give you our mind and commit our focus on you. As we focus on you, help us to focus on the things that matter most in life and to not worry about the rest. We pray this in Jesus' name. Amen."

NOTES

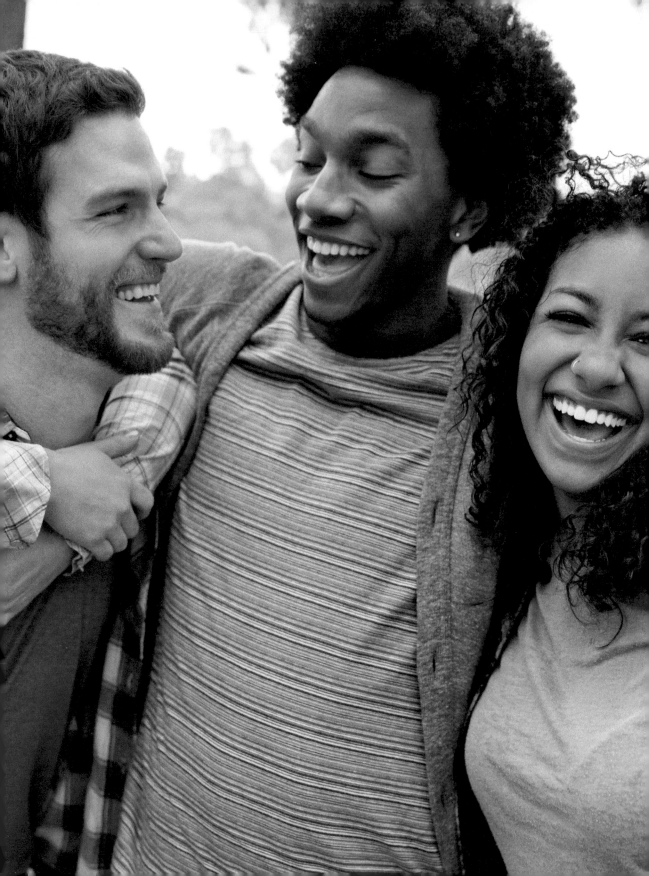

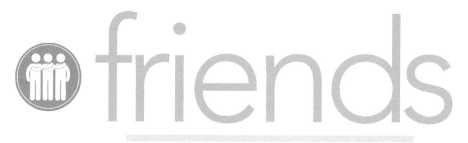

friends

ENCOURAGING *one* ANOTHER

> "Two people are better off
> than one, for they can help
> each other succeed."
> Ecclesiastes 4:9 (NLT)

As we learned last week when we studied Focus, one of the most important elements of achieving better health is sustaining change. We need support because we can't do it by our own sheer willpower. What makes The Daniel Plan unique is its "secret sauce" of community. By enlisting the help of friends, you'll discover not only accountability and support but the joy of community. We really are better together.

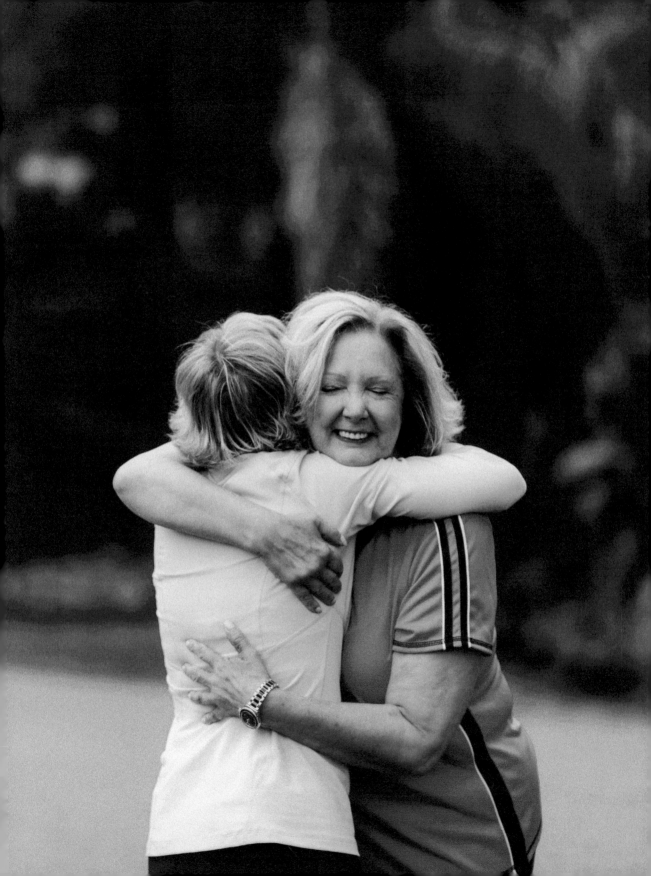

COMING
TOGETHER

Start by sharing and celebrating progress. Did anyone try the move of the week or a new recipe? Did anyone memorize a verse or learn something new? Use these questions to jump-start the conversation.

1 Share about a time you set a goal and a friend helped you achieve it. What happened? What did they do to help? How did the experience impact your friendship?

_____

_____

_____

2 Do you agree or disagree with the statement below? Why or why not? Tell about a time you experienced this in your own life.

_____

_____

_____

"When we are close and connected, experiencing love and acceptance, being cared for and supported, we are much more likely to choose healthy behaviors."
- The Daniel Plan -

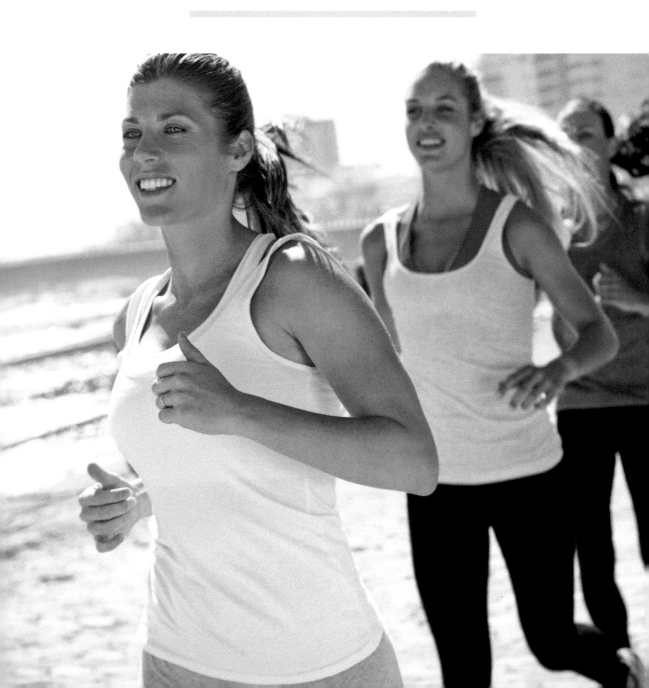

LEARNING
TOGETHER

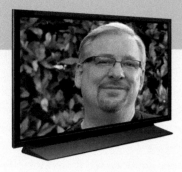

A MESSAGE FROM

Pastor Rick

Watch the video together. Use the following outline to take notes. The answers are in the appendix if you need them.

1 God designed us to _____ in relationships. We are always better together.

> » In order to follow through with a big challenge, you need God's power and you need a partner.

"Two are better than one, because they have a good return for their labor: If either of them falls down, one can help the other up."
Ecclesiastes 4:9–10 (NIV)

"So then, let us be always seeking the ways which lead to peace and the ways in which we can support one another."
Romans 14:19 (NJB)

2 You can summarize the purpose of life in two sentences. Love _____ with all your heart. Love your _____ as yourself.

> » If I want permanent change in my life, I must fill my life with love.

> » Love is the most powerful force in the universe, because God is love.

"Don't just pretend that you love others: really love them ... Love each other with brotherly affection and take delight in honoring each other."
Romans 12:9-10 (LB)

3 There are four ways that we demonstrate love for one another.

» We must _____ to each other.

» Be willing to _____ from each other.

» We need to be able to _____ with each other.

» We need to _____ each other.

"Instead, speaking the truth in love, growing in every way more and more like Christ."
Ephesians 4:15 (NLT)

"Be kind and compassionate to one another, forgiving each other, just as in Christ God forgave you."
Ephesians 4:32 (NIV)

"Our social circles influence our health even more than our DNA. If our friends have healthy habits, then we probably will too."
- Dr. Mark Hyman -

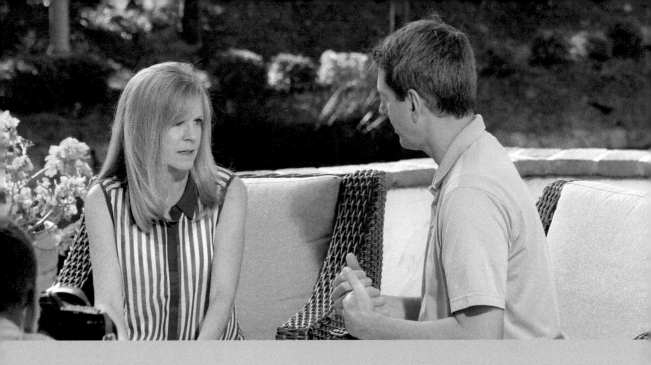

AN INTERVIEW WITH

Pastor Steve Willis

If our children aren't being all that God wants them to be, if they're not achieving what they could, just because they aren't eating the right foods, then that's a _____ issue.

» Poor nutrition impacts a child's ability to concentrate in school and leads to early death or disability in adults.

» If the church can support each other in our efforts to become healthier, we would all find greater time and energy to serve God and our communities.

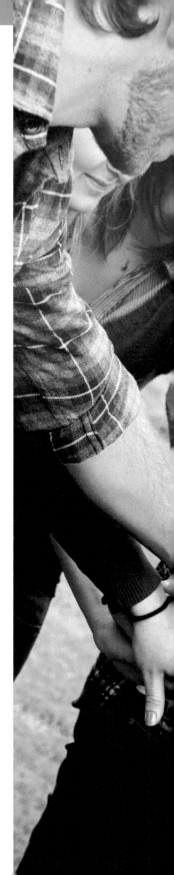

5 The Daniel Plan offers a _____ _____ message.

» When you speak the truth in love, people are more open to accept it.

6 If you want to make changes in your life, especially in the areas of health and nutrition, hang out with people who _____ _____.

» Community is what spurs us on to making the changes that we really need.

» You are more likely to be influenced by the friends you spend time with than by your parents' genetics.

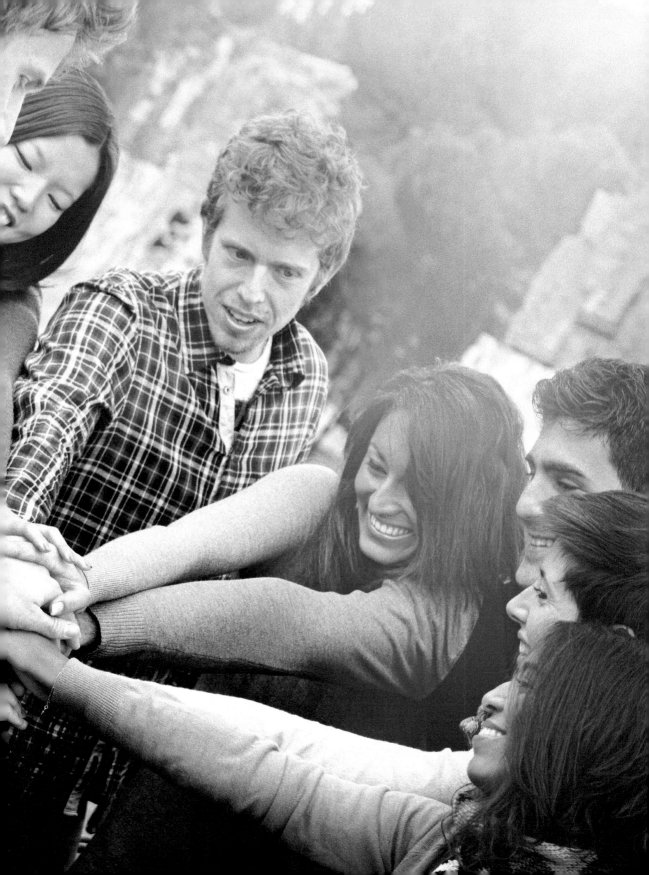

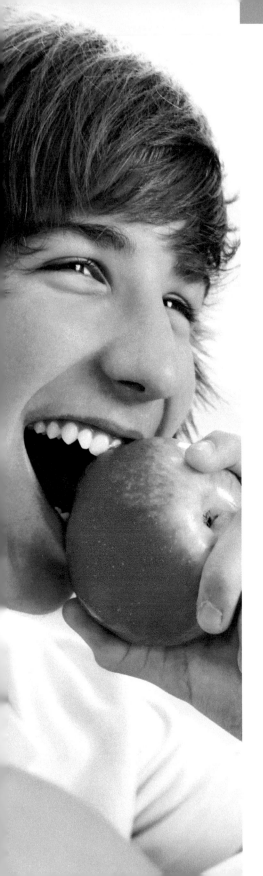

GROWING
TOGETHER

In this section, discuss what you learned from the video teaching. There's no single "right answer" here—just a chance for people to share their stories and listen to each other.

1 Pastor Rick talked about four keys to demonstrating love for one another: listen to each other, learn from one another, level with each other, and liberate each other. Why are these so challenging for us to do? Which one, to you, feels the most loving when you receive it?

_____

_____

_____

_____

_____

_____

2 In this week's video, Pastor Steve told a story of how improving nutrition and exercise in community had a profound result. Discuss some options that could work with your friends, family, or community?

_____

_____

_____

_____

3 Share about a time when you had a positive conversation about health and fitness—or actually worked with someone, to improve your health. What happened as a result?

_____

_____

_____

_____

_____

In the next section, called Better Together, we will offer you practical next steps to explore what you have learned and apply it to your everyday life. This week we will offer next steps for The Daniel Plan Friends Essential, along with Food and Fitness tips and recommendations.

BETTER
TOGETHER

Let's get practical—and put what we're learning into action. This week, we're talking about Friends, so be sure you're reaching out to do things together! We also have Food and Fitness activities for you to choose from.

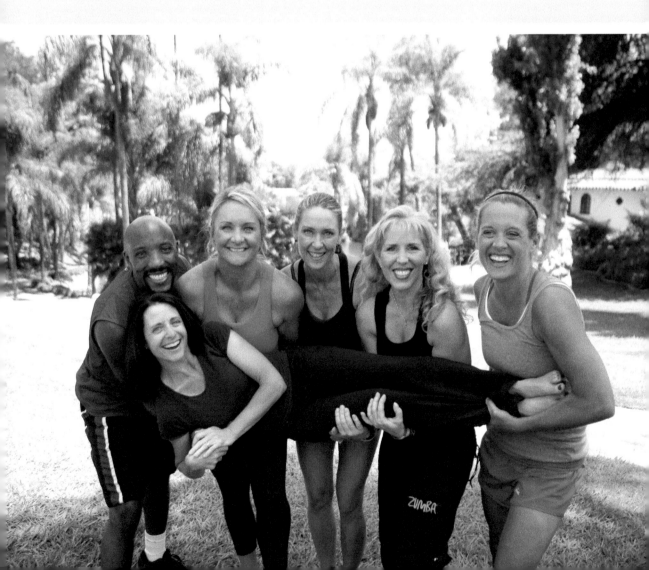

FRIENDS NEXT STEPS

Friends are the "secret sauce" of The Daniel Plan. Set up a time to get together with one or two friends this week—for a healthy meal, a hike or workout, or just to talk and pray together. Tell the group what you're planning, and then next week, share what happened.

How has this group helped you on your journey toward better health? Take some time right now to express your thankfulness and appreciation to the group for the ways they've supported you.

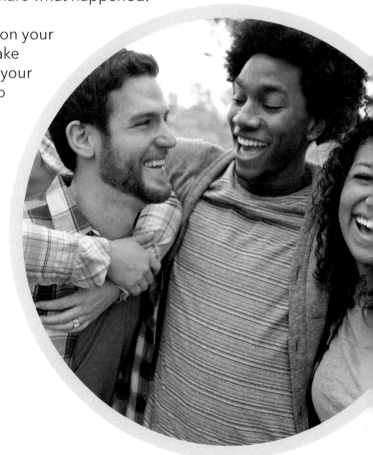

Everybody needs a buddy.

Here are a few tips and suggested activities to help you move forward on your journey toward health. **Check one or two boxes** next to the options you'd like to try–choose what works for you! You'll find helpful bonus material on the video.

FOOD NEXT STEPS

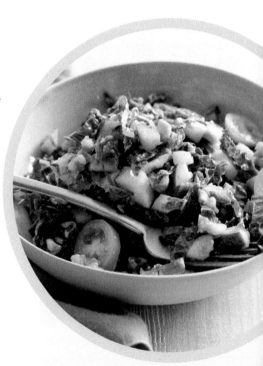

☐ **Food Tip of the Week:** Learn to shop the perimeter of the grocery store. This is where you will find all the whole foods. Visit your local farmers market for fresh in-season fruits and vegetables.

☐ **Recipe of the Week:** Bored with your salads? This week you will learn how to make a great salad. Just click The Daniel Plan Recipe of the Week button on the screen, scan the QR code, or go to danielplan.com/videos/great-salad.

☐ **Group Activity of the Week:** Watch the video to learn how to create a Daniel Plan style salad bar. Plan a time for the group to get together and have each person bring a different ingredient to make an amazing salad (or better yet, shop together!). Enjoy this healthy meal together–perhaps right before your next regularly scheduled meeting.

FITNESS NEXT STEPS

☐ **Fitness Tip of the Week:** Think about what motivates you to move your body and live well. What is your deeper reason for exercising on a regular basis? In other words, "What is your why?" Take some time this week to write down your "why" on a 3 x 5 card or your smartphone, and then discuss it with your group next week.

☐ **Move of the Week:** Watch the one-minute Daniel Plan Move of the Week video (just click The Daniel Plan Move of the Week button on the screen). Try it right now with the group, use the QR code, or go to danielplan.com/videos/move-of-the-week to watch it on your own.

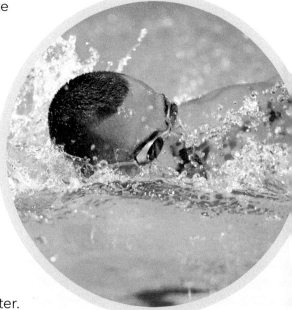

☐ **Group Activity of the Week:** Plan an outing with other group members this week. Put it on your calendar. Looking for a new idea? Go to the beach or a pool (at your local YMCA if it's winter), and try doing some "water aerobics" moves—even just walking in waist-high water.

EACH WEEK

We highly encourage you to read a few chapters of *The Daniel Plan: 40 Days to a Healthier Life* as you go through this study. This week, read Chapter 7: Friends.

PRAYING
TOGETHER

Because our efforts at living healthier are strengthened by prayer, we end each meeting with prayer and encourage group members to pray for each other during the week.

This week, take the exercise you did in the Friends Next Step of the Better Together section, where you expressed gratitude to the group for their support. Turn that same thankfulness and gratitude toward God. Thank him for the friends in your group, and outside the group, who support your efforts to be healthy. Let group members pray one- or two-sentence prayers of gratitude for friends. Then, the leader can close with the following benediction from Pastor Rick:

"God, our desire is that we will become people who are healthy, but more important than that, people who have a heart for you, who love you with all our hearts, love our neighbors, love everybody else as we love ourselves. We believe that your Word teaches us the truth about love. Help us to become loving people. Help us to practice listening, learning, liberating and even standing with that person when everything goes wrong. Help us to level with each other in truth, but help us to always do it out of love, not out of frustration, not out of fear, not out of guilt, not out of pressure. Help us to treat each other, Jesus, the way you treat us. I pray this in Jesus' name. Amen."

NOTES

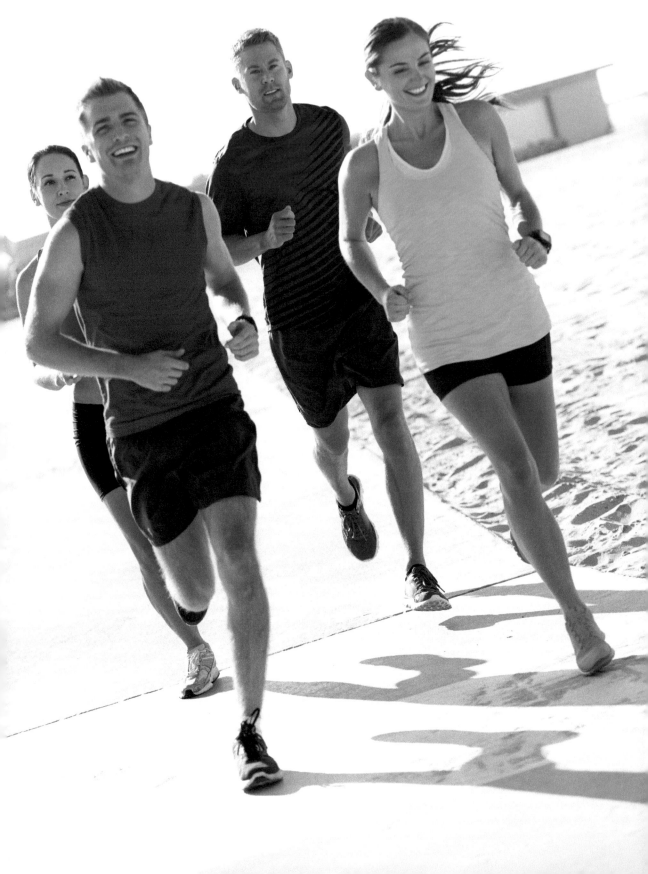

living the lifestyle

FULFILLING *your* PURPOSE

> "Anyone who belongs to Christ
> is a new person. The past is
> forgotten, and everything is new."
> 2 Corinthians 5:17 (CEV)

What sometimes seems like the end of a journey is only the beginning. Now you have all the Essentials you need—and this is where your journey continues. By exercising your faith in God, making small but significant changes to your food and fitness habits, renewing your focus, and enlisting friends for accountability and support, you can find the power to fulfill God's purpose for your life. You now know that small changes do indeed lead to big results. You are equipped to sustain these positive changes over the long haul.

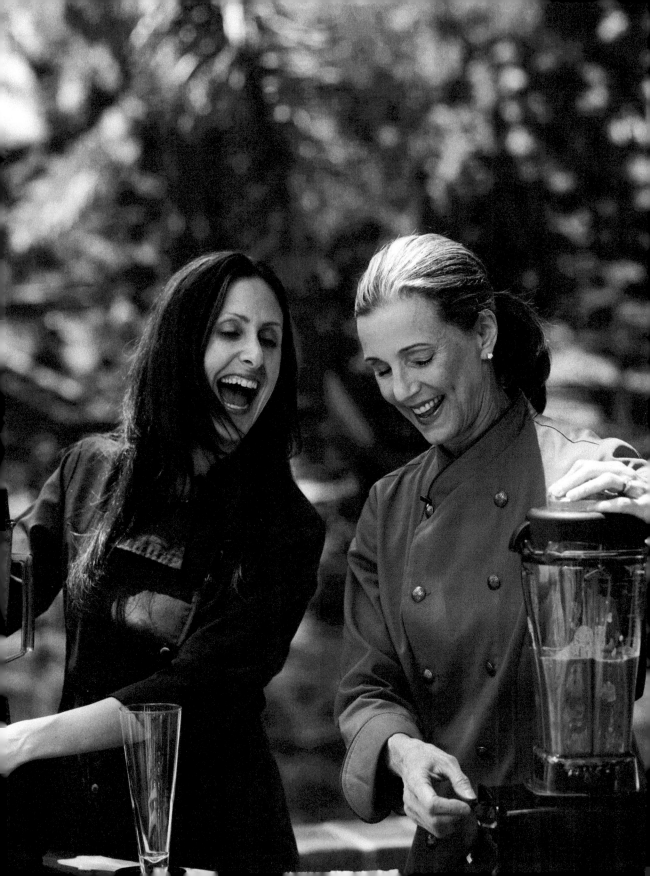

COMING
TOGETHER

Begin by celebrating progress: Did anyone try the move of the week or a new recipe? Memorize a verse? Use these questions to get people talking.

1 In which of the five Essentials—Faith, Food, Fitness, Focus, or Friends—have you seen the biggest change as a result of this study? Be specific—what was your "then" and what is your "now"?

_____

_____

_____

2 In your journey toward better health in all areas of your life, what has it meant to "bring in the good"?

_____

_____

_____

"If we focus on bringing in the good, enjoying the abundance of what God has given us, we will become stronger in body, mind, and spirit."
- The Daniel Plan -

LEARNING
TOGETHER

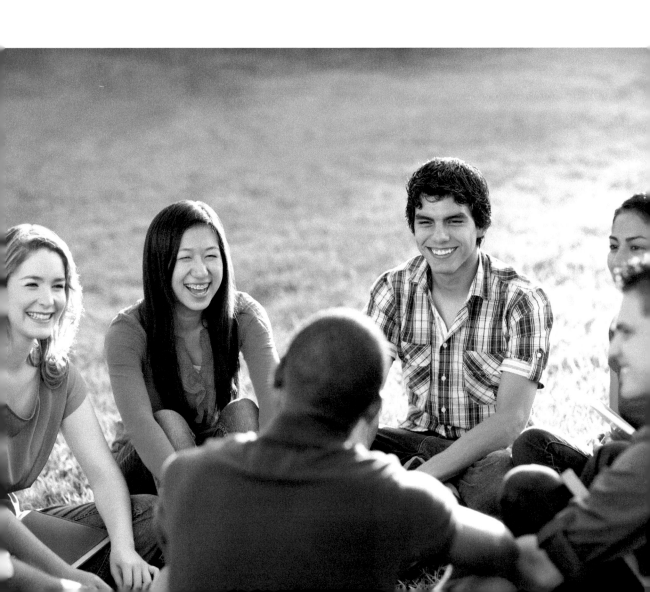

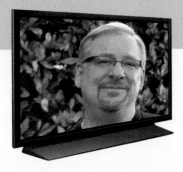

A MESSAGE FROM
Pastor Rick

Watch the video together. Use the following outline to take notes. The answers are in the appendix if you need them.

If you want to accomplish the goals that you have set for yourself, you have to make these strategies a priority in your life.

 1   We must remove all _____.

"Let us strip off anything that slows us down or holds us back … and let us run with patience the particular race that God has set before us."
Hebrews 12:1 (LB)

» The number one thing that keeps people from becoming what God wants them to be is their past.

"Forget the former things; do not dwell on the past."
Isaiah 43:18 (NIV)

"Forgetting the past and looking forward to what lies ahead, I press on to reach the end of the race."
Philippians 3:13–14 (NLT)

"Obstacles are what you see when you take your eye off the goal."
- Rick Warren -

2   We must remember the _____ and the _____.

>» Our primary reason for following The Daniel Plan is to bring glory to God.

>» The reward of living The Daniel Plan lifestyle is better physical health, more strength and energy, a sharper mind, deeper friendships, and a stronger faith.

3   We must _____ ourselves daily.

"We never become discouraged ... yet our spiritual being is renewed day after day."
2 Corinthians 4:16 (GNB)

"Lord, when doubts fill my mind, when my heart is in turmoil, quiet me and give me renewed hope and cheer."
Psalm 94:19 (LB)

>» Take time to be quiet and communicate with God every day.

>» When you begin to doubt yourself, remember three things: God's goodness yesterday, God's presence today, and God's promises for tomorrow.

4 We must _____ discouragement.

» Discouragement is an enemy of your goals.

"And let us not get tired of doing what is right, for after a while we will reap a harvest of blessing if we don't get discouraged and give up."
Galatians 6:9 (LB)

5 Finally, we must _____ on Christ.

» Willpower is NOT enough.

"For God is working in you, giving you the desire and the power to do what pleases him."
Philippians 2:13 (NLT)

"And I am sure that God who began the good work within you will keep right on helping you grow in his grace until his task within you is finally finished."
Philippians 1:6 (LB)

» Don't focus on failures. Focus on Christ.

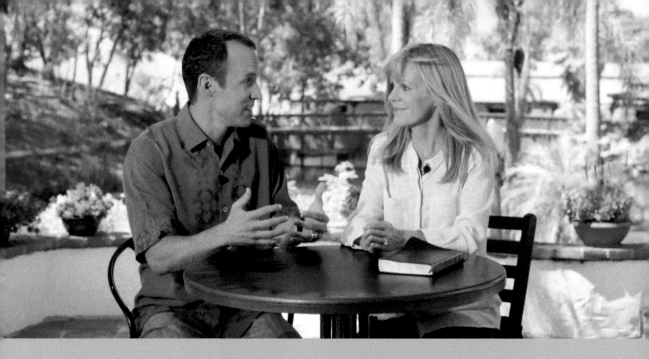

AN INTERVIEW WITH

Jimmy Peña Founder of Prayfit

  The Daniel Plan is about _____, not deprivation.

» Find healthy things you like doing and keep doing them.

» The goal is not to deprive, but to thrive.

Jesus said, "I came that they may have life and have it abundantly."
John 10:10b (ESV)

7 When we take it a _____ at a time, that makes all the difference in our lives.

» Continue exploring new foods and movement you enjoy.

» Repeating healthy actions leads to a changed mind and body.

8 It's not about perfection, it's about the _____.

» It's a process full of grace.

> *"My grace is sufficient for you, for my power is*
> *made perfect in weakness."*
> 2 Corinthians 12:9a (NIV)

"It's okay if you make mistakes.
If you get a little off-track, just make a U-turn."
- The Daniel Plan -

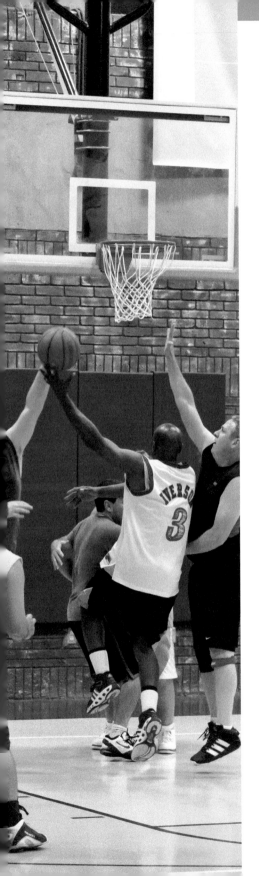

GROWING
TOGETHER

In this section, discuss the ideas you learned from the video teaching. There's no single "right answer" here, but simply some questions to get you thinking and sharing.

1 In the video, Pastor Rick shared five keys to sustaining your Daniel Plan journey: remove distractions, remember the reason and reward, renew ourselves, resist discouragement, and rely on Christ. Which of these was particularly significant for you? Why?

_____

_____

_____

_____

_____

_____

2 Pastor Rick challenged us to take five minutes somewhere in our day to simply be quiet, to renew our spirits with a few moments of calm. Is this a regular habit in your life? What barriers get in the way of making this a regular spiritual practice?

---

3 Jimmy Peña talked about healthy habits that come from practicing healthy behaviors. What are one or two "healthy habits" that you've developed as a result of this study? What is your plan for sustaining those habits going forward?

---

4 Jimmy and Dee talked about energy gains and energy drains. Share a few things that would add replenishment as you continue your Daniel Plan journey.

In the next section, called Better Together, we will offer you practical next steps to explore what you have learned and apply it to your everyday life. In this final week we will offer next steps for Living the Lifestyle, along with Food and Fitness tips and recommendations.

BETTER
TOGETHER

Let's get practical—and put what we're learning into action. This week, we're talking about Living the Lifestyle, so this is the time when everything you learned comes together so beautifully! We also have Food and Fitness activities for you to choose from.

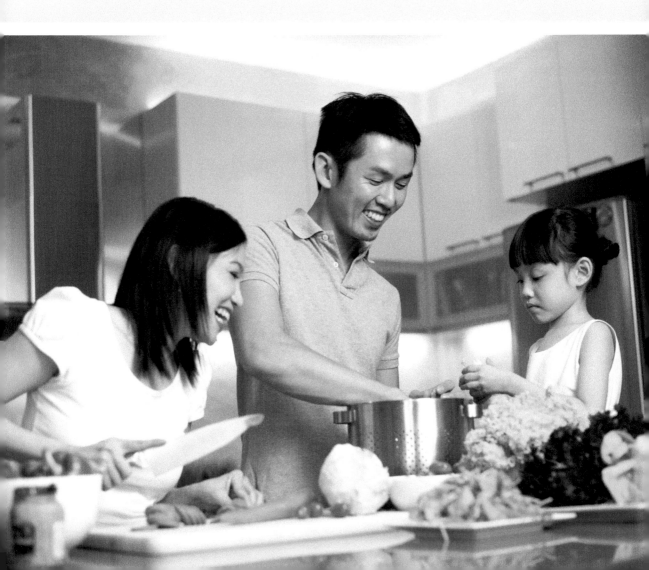

DANIEL PLAN NEXT STEPS

Take some time to celebrate what you have accomplished collectively as a group. What lasting changes have you made? How many pounds or inches have you lost as a group, for example? How, specifically, has your health improved—things like lower blood pressure, reduced or eliminated medications, spiritual renewal, etc.

_____

_____

What one next step do you need to take in order to keep on running the race set before you? What do you need to embrace or reject? Perhaps your next step is to lead a Daniel Plan group of your own. Visit danielplan.com/leadership for next steps.

_____

_____

Even though we are completing this small group study, continuing to live The Daniel Plan lifestyle is a lifelong process. How can this group help you continue in your journey toward greater health?

_____

_____

> "Failures aren't a setback.
> They are a setup for
> a comeback."
> – Dee Eastman -

EACH WEEK

Take a moment now to complete the 5 Essentials Survey (see appendix). Compare your score to day one. Share the results with the group and celebrate everything you have achieved over the last 40 days!

Here are a few tips and suggested activities to help you move forward on your journey toward health. **Check one or two boxes** next to the options you'd like to try–choose what works for you! You'll find helpful bonus material on the video.

FOOD NEXT STEPS

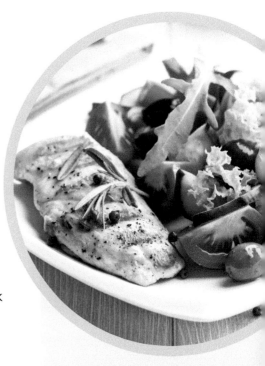

☐ **Food Tip of the Week:** Sometimes we mistake thirst for hunger. Drinking plenty of water is vital to overall health. Each day, you should drink half your body weight in ounces of water. For example, if you weigh 150 pounds, target drinking 75 ounces of fresh, filtered water daily.

☐ **Recipe of the Week:** Cooking chicken for dinner or just planning ahead helps you stay on track throughout the week. Just click The Daniel Plan Recipe of the Week button on the screen, scan the QR code, or go to danielplan.com/videos/cooking-chicken.

☐ **Group Activity of the Week:** Plan a healthy potluck dinner to celebrate your successes as a group. You might do a barbeque–try grilling some veggies and fruit to complement the meat you are cooking. For a simple approach, just have everyone bring different kinds of soup and salad.

FITNESS NEXT STEPS

- ☐ **Fitness Tip of the Week:** Be aware of statements that produce self-blame, shame, or guilt. If you miss an exercise session or were inactive for a short period of time, don't beat yourself up! Simply assess your lifestyle at the time, learn from it, and move forward. Maintaining an active, healthy lifestyle requires patience, persistence, and, most importantly, forgiveness. Focus on progress, not perfection.

- ☐ **Move of the Week:** Watch the one-minute Daniel Plan Move of the Week video (just click The Daniel Plan Move of the Week button on the screen). Try it right now with the group, use the QR code, or go to danielplan.com/videos/move-of-the-week to watch it on your own.

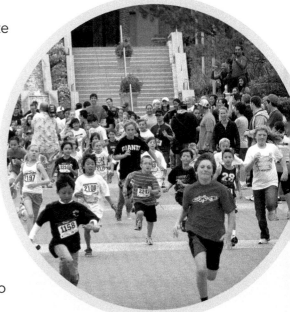

- ☐ **Group Activity of the Week:** Make plans to run or walk a 5K together. Have one or two people research local race options. From now until the race, get together with other group members to train.

You are almost finished reading *The Daniel Plan: 40 Days to a Healthier Life*. In this final week, read Chapter 8: Living the Lifestyle.
If you haven't already created your FREE Daniel Plan Health Profile, do it now at danielplan.com.

PRAYING
TOGETHER

Because our efforts at living healthier are strengthened by prayer, we end each meeting with prayer and encourage group members to pray for each other during the week.

A tradition in some churches is a call and response which goes like this: The leader says, "God is good" and the people respond, "All the time!" Then the leader says, "All the time" and the people respond, "God is good!" Use this (feel free to repeat it a few times) to open your prayer time with celebration! Then take some time to name some specific ways in which God has been good to you over the past six weeks of your Daniel Plan journey. Thank God for prayers that have been answered, new friendships that have developed, and new behaviors that have become lifelong healthy habits. After some time of praising God for his goodness, the leader can close with this benediction from Pastor Rick's message:

"Dear God, we were made for your purpose and you have a race that is unique to each of us. We want to make it to the finish line. We want our life to count, so forgive us for all those times we've gotten distracted. Help us to lay aside the distractions of life. Help us to resist discouragement. Help us to renew ourselves daily by spending time with you and just being quiet and learning the things that recharge our emotional batteries. Help us to rely on your power, do what you want us to do, and accomplish what you want us to accomplish. Most of all, Jesus, help us to remember how much you love us and to focus on you, to rely on you in every moment of life. Not just in our physical health but in our emotional, spiritual, relational, and mental health. We trust you and we expect you to help us in the days ahead and make it to the finish line in Jesus' name. Amen."

NOTES

APPENDIX

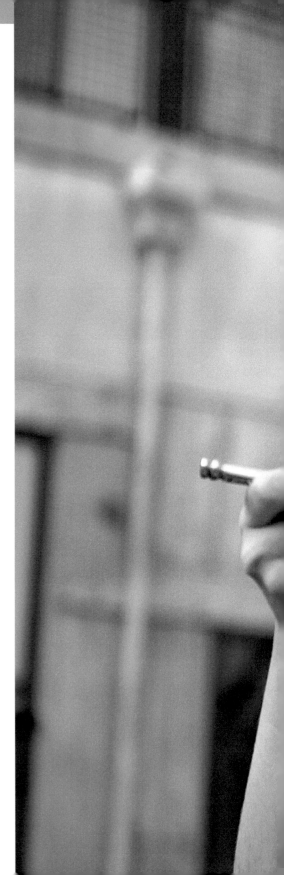

DANIEL PLAN RESOURCES

5 Essentials Survey

The Daniel Plan Plate

Top 10 Tips to Curb Your Cravings

SMALL GROUP RESOURCES

Group Guidelines

Frequently Asked Questions

Reading Plan for *The Daniel Plan: 40 Days to a Healthier Life*

Group Roster

Leadership Training 101

Daniel Plan Contributors

Acknowledgments

Answer Key

Disclaimer

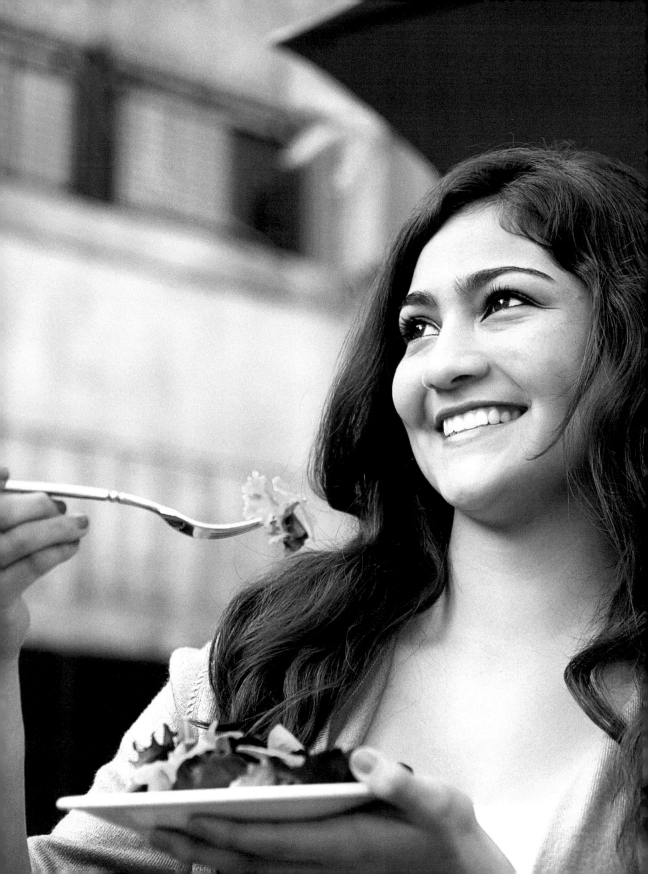

DANIEL PLAN RESOURCES

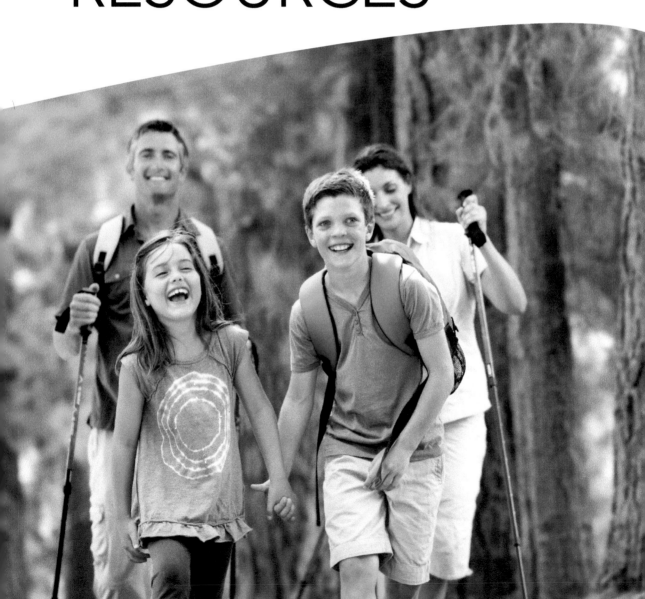

5 ESSENTIALS SURVEY

On a scale of 1-5, please use the following to rate your current status related to The Daniel Plan 5 Essentials. We'd encourage you to take this survey both at the beginning and end of the program.

FAITH	Very Dissatisfied	Dissatisfied	Neutral	Satisfied	Very Satisfied
Relationship with God	1	2	3	4	5
Sense of meaning and purpose in life	1	2	3	4	5
Spiritual practices: prayer, worship, meditation	1	2	3	4	5
Spiritual growth	1	2	3	4	5
Giving to others	1	2	3	4	5
Add up each column and enter your total Faith score:					

FOOD	Never	Rarely	Sometimes	Most of the time	Daily
I eat 7 or more servings of a variety of fruits and vegetables daily	1	2	3	4	5
I eat lean protein with every meal	1	2	3	4	5
I drink 1/2 my body weight in ounces each day	1	2	3	4	5
I choose healthy fats	1	2	3	4	5
I eat a healthy, nutritious breakfast	1	2	3	4	5
Add up each column and enter your total Food score:					

FITNESS HOW I FEEL ABOUT:	Very Dissatisfied	Dissatisfied	Neutral	Satisfied	Very Satisfied
My body (appearance/weight)	1	2	3	4	5
My cardiovascular endurance	1	2	3	4	5
My strength	1	2	3	4	5
My flexibility	1	2	3	4	5
My health	1	2	3	4	5
Add up each column and enter your total Fitness score:					

FOCUS	Very Dissatisfied	Dissatisfied	Neutral	Satisfied	Very Satisfied
Positive mental attitude	1	2	3	4	5
Achievement of personal goals	1	2	3	4	5
Peace of mind	1	2	3	4	5
Gratitude and thankfulness	1	2	3	4	5
Ability to handle mistakes or failures	1	2	3	4	5
Add up each column and enter your total Focus score:					

FRIENDS	Very Dissatisfied	Dissatisfied	Neutral	Satisfied	Very Satisfied
Relationship with my significant other	1	2	3	4	5
Relationships with my family	1	2	3	4	5
Relationship with my friends	1	2	3	4	5
Relationship with others (coworkers or neighbors)	1	2	3	4	5
My communication skills	1	2	3	4	5
Add up each column and enter your total Friends score:					

RESULTS

Congratulations! Now that you have completed your Daniel Plan Essentials survey, transfer your scores for each area of wellness (Faith, Food, Fitness, Friends and Focus) in the table below in the "My score" column. Next, read the following pages to get a better understanding of what your scores mean as well as learning about the stages of change and how to move forward with your program.

DAY 1		DAY 40	
	MY SCORE		MY SCORE
FAITH		FAITH	
FOOD		FOOD	
FITNESS		FITNESS	
FRIENDS		FRIENDS	
FOCUS		FOCUS	

20-25: Well done! If you scored between 20-25 points for a particular Daniel Plan Essential, your answers demonstrate you are aware of the importance of this area to your personal wellness and have developed healthy habits.

15-20: If you scored between 15-20 in one or more of your Daniel Plan Essentials, your health and wellness practices are going well, but you may have room for some improvement. Identify the statements you are unsatisfied with and begin to review tips and strategies in *The Daniel Plan: 40 Days to a Healthier Life* and this group study to help improve your score the next time you take this survey.

10-15: If you scored between 10-15 in one or more of your Daniel Plan Essentials, this may be an ideal area in which to begin to focus your attention and set specific goals.

Scores below 10: If you scored below 10 in one or more of your Daniel Plan Essentials, it's time to focus your attention on making some changes. Identify all statements on which you may have scored yourself 1 or 2 and begin to consider your interest in improving these areas. We also would encourage you to read Stages of Change on our website, danielplan .com/stages-of-change/, to help you begin to make small steps toward improving in this area.

To help you narrow your focus, identify the #1 Daniel Plan Essential you would most like to improve or change: (Check one answer)

- ☐ Faith
- ☐ Food
- ☐ Fitness
- ☐ Friends
- ☐ Focus

Select one statement that best describes your readiness to make the lifestyle change in the Essential selected above.

- ☐ "I'm just not interested in working on changes in this area at the moment."
- ☐ "I'm thinking about improving this area of my life in the next few months."
- ☐ "I'm planning to begin to work on this area in the next 40 days."
- ☐ "I am ready now to start working on this area of my life."
- ☐ "I have been actively working on improving my life in this area over at least the last six months."

THE DANIEL PLAN PLATE

The Daniel Plan gives an easy guideline to use for any meal:

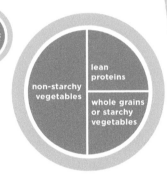

- ☐ 50 percent non-starchy veggies
- ☐ 25 percent healthy animal or vegetable protein
- ☐ 25 percent healthy starch or whole grains
- ☐ Side of low-sugar (low-glycemic) fruit
- ☐ Water or caffeine-free herbal teas with lemon

Here are some great choices to start with:

NON-STARCHY VEGGIES	PROTEIN	STARCH OR GRAIN	LOW-GLYCEMIC FRUIT
Asparagus	Beans	Beets	Apples
Bell peppers	Beef	Brown/black rice	Blackberries
Broccoli	Chicken	Carrots	Blueberries
Cauliflower	Eggs	Buckwheat	Gogi berries
Collard greens	Halibut	Green peas	Grapefruit
Cucumbers	Lentils	Corn	Plums
Green beans	Nuts	Quinoa	Kiwi
Kale	Salmon	Sweet potatoes	Nectarines
Spinach	Seeds	Turnips	Peaches
Zucchini	Turkey	Winter squash	Raspberries

TOP 10 TIPS TO CURB YOUR CRAVINGS

1. Avoid your triggers: The reality is that you crave what you eat, so as you make healthier choices, your old cravings will weaken. Certain situations can sabotage your weight loss efforts. For example, going to the movies can ignite your brain's emotional memory centers and make you feel like you need an extra-large tub of popcorn. Identify the people, places, and things that trigger your cravings and plan ahead to avoid making an unhealthy choice. For example, take a healthy snack to the movies so you are not tempted to buy popcorn. This will save you money too!

2. Balance your blood sugar: Research studies indicate that low blood sugar levels are associated with lower overall blood flow to the brain, which can jeopardize your ability to make good decisions. To keep your blood sugar stable, eat a nutritious breakfast with protein, such as eggs, a protein shake, or nut butters. Plan to eat smaller, more frequent meals throughout the day. Also, avoid eating two to three hours before bedtime.

3. Eliminate sugar, artificial sweeteners, and refined carbs: It's best to go cold turkey. Eliminate refined sugars, sodas, fruit juices, and artificial sweeteners from your diet, as these can trigger cravings. Many doctors believe that sugar is the primary cause of obesity, high blood pressure, heart disease, and diabetes. The latest statistics reveal that the average American consumes 130 pounds of sugar a year!

4. Eat SLOW carb, not LOW carb: Eat carbohydrates that don't spike your blood sugar. Choose high fiber carbs that keep you fuller longer and help reduce your sugar cravings. You can increase your fiber intake by eating vegetables, fruits, beans, and whole grains. Fiber will assist weight loss because it fills up your stomach and helps you moderate your portions. Carbohydrates are essential to good health and are not the enemy. Bad carbohydrates such as simple sugars and refined products are the ones to avoid.

5. Drink more water: Sometimes hunger is disguised as dehydration. When you are dehydrated, your body will increase your hunger level in an attempt to get more water to rehydrate. Try drinking a glass of water before your meals to make you feel fuller and thus moderate your food intake.

6. Make protein 25 percent of your diet: Protein fills you up and keeps you satisfied longer. It also regulates your blood sugar and makes your body release appetite-suppressing hormones.

7. Manage your stress: Stress triggers hormones that activate cravings. Chronic stress has been associated with obesity, addiction, anxiety, depression, Alzheimer's disease, heart disease, and cancer. Adopt a daily stress management program that includes deep breathing exercises, prayer, and other relaxation techniques.

8. Follow the 90/10 Rule: Give yourself a break. Make great food choices 90 percent of the time, and allow yourself margin to enjoy some of your favorite foods on occasion. This way you won't feel deprived, and you will avoid bingeing on something you'll regret later.

9. Get moving: Research shows that physical activity can curb cravings. Plan out your exercise for the week and schedule it on your calendar. Make the commitment to yourself just like any other important meeting or appointment.

10. Get seven to eight hours of sleep a night: Sleep deprivation can increase cravings. Check out our tips for healthy sleep habits on danielplan. com.

"Truly, what you put on your fork dictates whether you are sick or well, slim or fat, depleted or energized."

– Dr. Mark Hyman

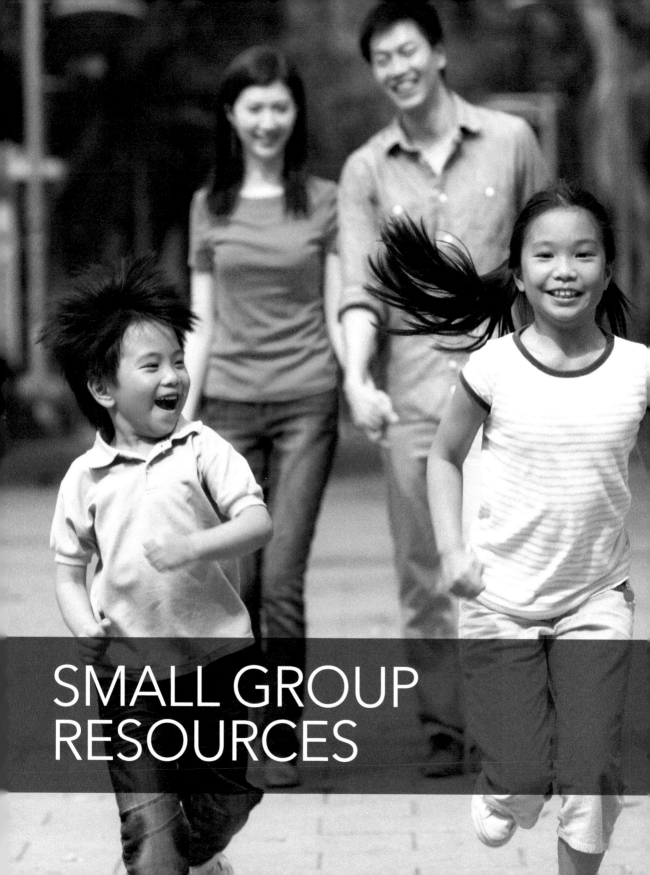

SMALL GROUP
RESOURCES

GROUP GUIDELINES

OUR VALUES	
Group Attendance	To give priority to the group meeting. We will call or email if we will be late or absent.
Save Environment	To help create a safe place where people can be heard and feel loved.
Respect Differences	To be gentle and gracious to people with different spiritual maturity, personal opinions, or personalities. Remember we are all works in progress!
Confidentiality	To keep anything that is shared strictly confidential and within the group, and to avoid sharing information about those outside the group.
Encouragement for Growth	We want to spiritually multiply our life by serving others with our God-given gifts.
Rotating Hosts/ Leaders and Home	To encourage different people to host the group in their homes, and to rotate the responsibility of facilitating each meeting.

Refreshments/mealtimes _____

Child care _____

When we will meet (day of week) _____

Where we will meet (place) _____

We will begin at (time) _____ and end at _____

We will do our best to have some or all of us attend a worship service together.

Our primary worship service time will be _____

FAQs

What do we do on the first night of our group?
Like all fun things in life—have a party! A "get to know you" gathering is a great way to launch a new study. Review the Group Guidelines (found earlier in the appendix) and share the names of a few friends you can invite to join you. But most importantly, have fun before your study time begins.

Where do we find new members for our group?
We encourage you to pray with your group and then brainstorm a list of people from work, church, your neighborhood, your children's school, family, the gym, and so on. Then have each group member invite several of the people on his or her list. Another good strategy is to ask church leaders to make an announcement or put an insert in the weekend bulletin.

No matter how you find members, it's vital that you stay open to new people joining your group. All groups tend to go through healthy attrition—the result of moves, releasing new leaders, ministry opportunities, and so forth—and if the group gets too small, it could be at risk of shutting down. If you and your group stay open, you'll be amazed at the people God sends your way. The next person just might become a friend for life. You never know!

How long will this group meet?
Once you come to the end of this six-week study, we encourage you to continue meeting together and stay committed to your Daniel Plan journey. You can get more resources at danielplan.com.

What if this group is not working for us?
This isn't uncommon. This could be the result of a personality conflict, life stage difference, geographical distance, level of spiritual maturity, or any number of things. Relax. Pray for God's direction, and at the end of this six-week study, decide whether to continue with this group or find another. You don't buy the first car you look at or marry the first person you date and

the same goes with a group. Don't drop out before the six weeks are up—
God might have something to teach you!

Who is the leader?

Most groups have an official leader. But ideally, the group will mature and
members will rotate the leadership of meetings. We have discovered that
healthy groups rotate hosts/leaders and homes on a regular basis. This
model ensures that all members grow, give their unique contribution, and
develop their gifts. This study guide and the Holy Spirit can keep things on
track even when you rotate leaders. Christ has promised to be in your midst
as you gather. Ultimately, God is your leader each step of the way.

How do we handle the child care needs in our group?

Since this can be a sensitive issue, handle this discussion with extra care.
We suggest that you empower the group to openly brainstorm solutions.
You may try one option that works for a while and then adjust over time.
Our favorite approach is for adults to meet in the living room or dining
room and share the cost of a babysitter (or two) who can be with the kids
in a different part of the house. In this way, parents don't have to be away
from their children all evening when their children are too young to be left
at home.

A second option is to use one home for the kids and a second home
(close by or a phone call away) for the adults. A third idea is to rotate the
responsibility of providing a lesson or care for the children either in the
same home or in another home nearby. This can be an incredible blessing
for kids. Finally, the most common idea is to decide that you need to have a
night to invest in your spiritual lives individually or as a couple, and to make
your own arrangements for child care. No matter what decision the group
makes, the best approach is to dialogue openly about the solution.

READING PLAN

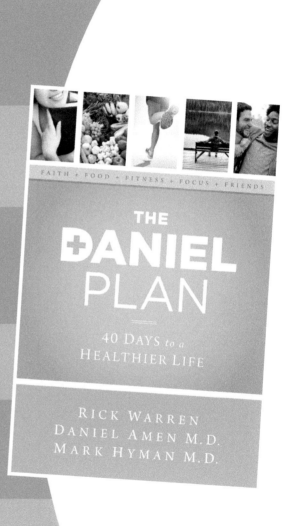

WEEK 1
Chapter 1: How It All Began
Chapter 2: The Essentials
Chapter 3: Faith

WEEK 2
Chapter 4: Food
Chapter 10: 40-Day Meal Plan

WEEK 3
Chapter 5: Fitness
Chapter 9: Daniel Strong
40-Day Fitness Challenge

WEEK 4
Chapter 6: Focus

WEEK 5
Chapter 7: Friends

WEEK 6
Chapter 8: Living the Lifestyle

GROUP ROSTER

NAME	ADDRESS	PHONE	EMAIL	OTHER

LEADERSHIP 101

Congratulations! You have responded to the call to help shepherd Jesus' flock. There are few other tasks in the family of God that surpass the contribution you will be making. As you prepare to lead, whether it is one session or the entire series, here are a few thoughts to keep in mind. We encourage you to read these and review them with each new discussion leader before he or she leads.

1. Remember that you are not alone. God knows everything about you, and he knew that you would be asked to lead your group. Remember that it is common for all good leaders to feel that they are not ready to lead. Moses, Solomon, Jeremiah, and Timothy–they all were reluctant to lead. God promises, "Never will I leave you; never will I forsake you" (Hebrews 13:5). Whether you are leading for one evening, for several weeks, or for a lifetime, you will be blessed as you serve.

2. Don't try to do it alone. Pray right now for God to help you build a healthy leadership team. If you can enlist a co-leader to help you lead the group, you will find your experience to be much richer. This is your chance to involve as many people as you can in building a healthy group. All you have to do is call and ask people to help; you'll be surprised at the response.

3. Just be yourself. If you won't be you, who will? God wants you to use your unique gifts and temperament. Don't try to do things exactly like another leader; do them in a way that fits you! Just admit it when you don't have an answer, and apologize when you make a mistake. Your group will love you for it, and you'll sleep better at night!

4. Prepare for your meeting ahead of time. Review the session, and write down your responses to each question. Pay special attention to exercises that ask group members to do something other than engage in discussion. These exercises will help your group live what the Bible teaches, not just talk about it. Be sure you understand how an exercise works, and bring any necessary supplies (such as paper and pens) to your meeting. If the exercise employs one of the resources in the appendix, be sure to look it over ahead of time so you'll know how it works.

5. Pray for your group members by name. Before you begin your session, go around the room in your mind and pray for each member by name. You may want to review the prayer list at least once a week. Ask God to use your time together to touch the heart of every person uniquely. Expect God to lead you to whomever he wants you to encourage or challenge in a special way.

6. When you ask a question, be patient. Someone will eventually respond. Sometimes people need a moment or two of silence to think about the question, and if silence doesn't bother you, it won't bother anyone else. After someone responds, affirm the response with a simple "thanks" or "good job." Then ask, "How about somebody else?" or "Would someone who hasn't shared like to add anything?" Be sensitive to new people or reluctant members who aren't ready to participate yet. If you give them a safe setting, they will open up over time.

7. Provide transitions between questions. When guiding the discussion, always read aloud the transitional paragraphs and the questions. Ask the group if anyone would like to read the paragraph or Bible passage. Don't call on anyone, but ask for a volunteer, and then be patient until someone begins. Be sure to thank the person who reads aloud.

8. Break up into small groups each week, or they won't stay. If your group has more than seven people, we strongly encourage you to have the group gather sometimes in discussion circles of three or four people during the GROWING TOGETHER section of the study. With a greater opportunity to talk in a small circle, people will connect more with the study, apply more quickly what they're learning, and ultimately get more out of it. A small circle also encourages a quiet person to participate and tends to minimize the effects of a more vocal or dominant member. It can also help people feel more loved in your group. When you gather again at the end of the section, you can have one person summarize the highlights from each circle.

Small circles are also helpful during prayer time. People who are not accustomed to praying aloud will feel more comfortable trying it with just two or three others. Also, prayer requests won't take as much time, so circles will have more time to actually pray. When you gather back with the whole group, you can have one person from each circle briefly update everyone on the prayer requests.

9. Rotate facilitators weekly. At the end of each meeting, ask the group who should lead the following week. Let the group help select your weekly facilitator. You may be perfectly capable of leading each time, but you will help others grow in their faith and gifts if you give them opportunities to lead.

10. One final challenge (for new or first-time leaders): Before your first opportunity to lead, look up each of the five passages listed below. Read each one as a devotional exercise to help equip you with a shepherd's heart. If you do this, you will be more than ready for your first meeting.

Matthew 9:36
1 Peter 5:2–4
Psalm 23
Ezekiel 34:11–16
1 Thessalonians 2:7–8, 11–12

DANIEL PLAN CONTRIBUTORS

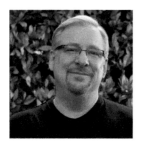

Rick Warren, D. Min. founded Saddleback Church in 1980 and now more than 120,000 people call Saddleback their church home. Pastor Rick is an internationally recognized author. His book, *The Purpose Driven Life*, has sold more than thirty million copies in English, and is published in over 100 languages.

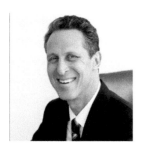

Mark Hyman, M.D. has dedicated his career to identifying and addressing the root causes of chronic illness through a whole-systems medicine approach known as Functional Medicine. He is a family physician, a four-time *New York Times* bestselling author, and an internationally recognized leader in his field.

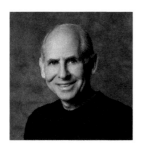

Daniel Amen, M.D. is a physician, Distinguished Fellow of the American Psychiatric Association, neuroscientist, and eight-time *New York Times* bestselling author. Dr. Amen's extensive research and innovative approach to optimizing the brain has helped millions of people worldwide.

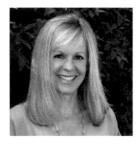

Dee Eastman, B.S. Health Sciences is the founding director for The Daniel Plan that helped over 15,000 people lose 260,000 pounds in the first year alone. Dee's background in corporate wellness and ministry has fueled her passion to help people transform their health while drawing closer to God. She coauthored a Bible study curriculum that has sold more than 3 million copies.

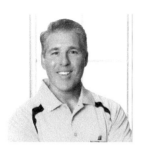

Sean Foy, B.S. Exercise Physiology, M.A. Marriage and Family Therapy is an internationally renowned authority on fitness, weight management, and healthy living, and has spent the last 20 years cracking the code to make fitness work. As an author, exercise physiologist, and speaker, Sean has earned the reputation as "America's Fast Fitness Expert."

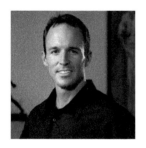

Jimmy Peña, M.S. Clinical Exercise Physiology is an author, exercise physiologist, and the founder of PrayFit. He has been the exercise physiologist to Tyler Perry, Mario Lopez, and LL Cool J, and was coauthor of the *New York Times* bestseller, *Extra Lean* by Mario Lopez. Jimmy is a long-standing member of The Daniel Plan Board of Advisors.

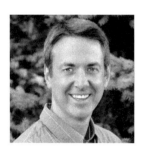

Steve Willis, Ed. D, Ph.D. is an author and lead pastor of First Baptist Church of Kenova, West Virginia. His passion for health led him to help the people of Huntington, West Virginia recover from being the most obese community in the nation. Steve is best known for his role on ABC's Emmy-winning mini-series *Jamie Oliver's Food Revolution.*

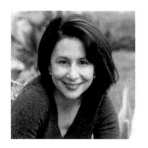

April O'Neil, B.A. Organizational Leadership is a writer and holistic health coach. Her corporate leadership experience combined with her passion to help people heal have become the cornerstone of her contributions. As the communications specialist for The Daniel Plan, she oversees a number of strategic initiatives including the weekly blog, website, and social media venues.

ACKNOWLEDGMENTS

From Dee Eastman, Director of The Daniel Plan

We are most grateful to Pastor Steve Willis, Keri Wyatt Kent, and Allen White for the creativity each of you poured into this study. Thank you for investing into this resource for our extended Daniel Plan Community and for bringing your passion for healthy living to the overall flow and design of this guide and video.

April O'Neil, your contribution in overseeing the entire development of this project was clearly driven by your passion for The Daniel Plan and your desire for people to begin healing. Your heart for life transformation and practical knowledge of the Essentials helped to shape the reader's experience.

With deep gratitude, we want to thank Kathrine Lee and Brian Williams for offering their valuable insight to the program and highlighting the most powerful principles for this study. The life coaching wisdom you imparted guided the best progression of next steps from week to week.

To our Daniel Plan Signature Chefs, Jenny Ross and Sally Cameron, thank you for teaching us how to cook food that loves us back! Your meal plans, food demos, and delicious recipes are an amazing complement to the program and will inspire people to get back in the kitchen.

Our community of fitness experts and instructors have infused their passion into the Fitness Essential, encouraging people to just take one step in the right direction. Thank you for your heart to serve and help people get moving toward better health.

To everyone who told their story—we applaud your courage to share your ups and downs. Your story will be a blessing to others, and encourage them to join The Daniel Plan and begin a journey of their own.

The creative impact of our video team brought The Daniel Plan to life on screen. We are most grateful to the leadership and collaboration of the production teams led by Josh Hailey and Frank Baker. The visual story you created provides an engaging way to learn and follow The Daniel Plan.

Buddy Owens—we can't thank you enough for all you have poured into this project; your contributions are significant and you are a delight to work with. To John Raymond and the entire Zondervan team—thank you for believing that this study has the potential to change lives. We appreciate your overall direction and supporting us through the process.

It is our prayer that you and your small group are deeply blessed by doing this study together. May God shine his light brightly on you and pour inspiration and motivation into your everyday life.

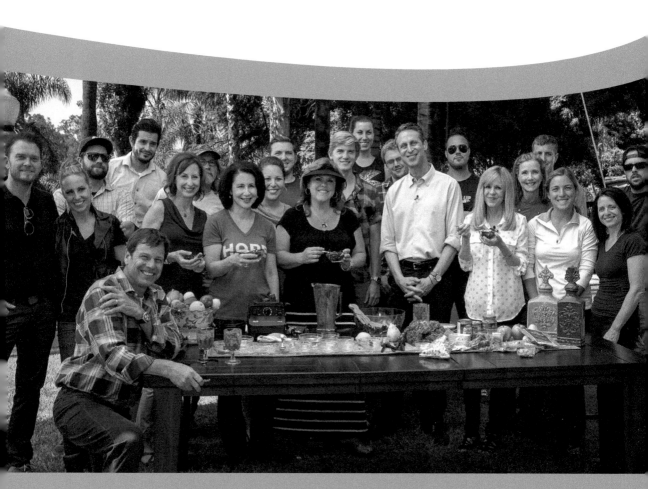

ANSWER KEY

Session 1–Faith

From Pastor Rick

1. broken
2. walking, acceptance,
   Spirit of God, faith,
   good, succeed, love

From Jimmy Peña

3. Faith
4. perfect
5. service

Session 2–Food

From Pastor Rick

1. overweight
2. body
3. caretaker

From Dr. Hyman

4. energy, instructions
5. labels
6. brain, protein, regular,
   liquid-sugar
7. quality

Session 3–Fitness

From Pastor Rick

1. purify, sanctify
2. physically
3. protect
4. motivation
5. worship, stewardship

From Sean Foy

6. do
7. emotion

Session 4–Focus

From Pastor Rick

1. plan
2. distractions
3. choice
4. deadline

From Dr. Amen

5. behavior
6. true
7. feel

Session 5–Friends

From Pastor Rick

1. thrive
2. God, neighbor
3. listen, learn,
   level, liberate

From Pastor Steve

4. moral
5. grace-filled
6. get it

Session 6–Living the Lifestyle

From Pastor Rick

1. distractions
2. reason, reward
3. renew
4. resist
5. rely

From Jimmy Peña

6. abundance
7. step
8. process

DISCLAIMER

The Daniel Plan offers health, fitness, and nutritional information and is for educational purposes only. This book is intended to supplement, not replace, the professional medical advice, diagnosis, or treatment of health conditions from a trained health professional.

Please consult your physician or other healthcare professional before beginning or changing any health or fitness program to make sure that it is appropriate for your needs—especially if you are pregnant or have a family history of any medical concerns, illnesses, or risks.

If you have any concerns or questions about your health, you should always consult with a physician or other healthcare professional. Stop exercising immediately if you experience faintness, dizziness, pain, or shortness of breath at any time. Please do not disregard, avoid, or delay obtaining medical or health-related advice from your healthcare professional because of something you may have read in this guide.

THE **DANIEL** PLAN

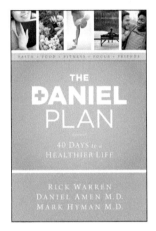

The Daniel Plan

40 Days to a Healthier Life

*Rick Warren D. Min., Daniel Amen M.D.,
Mark Hyman M.D.*

The Daniel Plan: 40 Days to a Healthier Life by Rick Warren, Dr. Daniel Amen, and Dr. Mark Hyman is an innovative approach to achieving a healthy lifestyle where people get better together by optimizing their health in the key areas of faith, food, fitness, focus, and friends. Within these five key life areas, readers are offered a multitude of resources and the foundation to get healthy. Ultimately, *The Daniel Plan* is about abundance, not deprivation, and this is why the plan is both transformational and sustainable.

The Daniel Plan Journal

40 Days to a Healthier Life

Rick Warren and the Daniel Plan Team

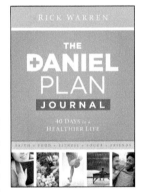

The Daniel Plan Journal is a practical and experiential tool filled with daily encouragement from Rick Warren and The Daniel Plan team. Scripture and inspirational quotes are also included. The journal was designed so users can record milestones related to all of The Daniel Plan Essentials: Faith, Food, Fitness, Focus, and Friends. This is an important element for those who want to maximize their potential to experience an all-around healthy lifestyle.

Available in stores and online!

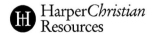

HarperChristian
Resources